PROFESSIONAL AND
ETHICAL ISSUES
IN NURSING

MW
NURS

PROFESSIONAL AND ETHICAL ISSUES IN NURSING

The Code of Professional Conduct

PHILIP BURNARD
MSc RGN RMN DipN CertEd RNT
Lecturer in Nursing Studies
School of Nursing Studies, University of Wales
College of Medicine, Cardiff

CHRISTINE M CHAPMAN
OBE BSc (Hons) MPhil SRN SCM RNT FRCN
Professor of Nursing Education,
Dean of the School of Nursing Studies,
University of Wales College of Medicine, Cardiff

An H M + M Nursing Publication

JOHN WILEY & SONS
Chichester · New York · Brisbane · Toronto · Singapore

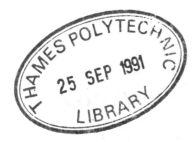

© John Wiley & Sons Ltd 1988

Reprinted 1990
Reprinted 1991

H M + M Publishers is an imprint of John Wiley & Sons Ltd,
Baffins Lane, Chichester, Sussex PO19 1UD, England

Library of Congress Cataloging in Publication Data

Burnard, Philip.
    Professional and ethical issues in nursing: the code of professional conduct /
Philip Burnard, Christine M. Chapman.
        p.   cm.—(An H M + M nursing publication)
    Bibliography: p.
    Includes index
    ISBN 0-471-92025-8 (pbk)
    1. Nursing ethics.   I. Chapman, Christine M.   II. Title.
    III. Series.
    [DNLM: 1. Ethics, Nursing.   WY 85 B963p]
    RT85.B87   1988
    174'.2—dc19
    DNLM/DLC
    for Library of Congress   88-14358 CIP

British Library Cataloguing in Publication Data

Burnard, Philip
    Professional and ethical issues in nursing: the Code of Professional Conduct.
    1. Medicine. Nursing. Ethical aspects
    I. Title   II. Chapman, Christine M. (Christine Muriel, *1927*–
    174'.2
    ISBN 0 471 92025 8 ✓

Typeset by Words&Spaces, Rowlands Castle, Hampshire, England
Printed and bound in Great Britain by
Biddles Ltd, Guildford and King's Lynn

Contents

Preface

The Nurses, Midwives and Health Visitor's Act 1979 gave power to the United Kingdom Central Council for Nursing, Midwifery and Health Visiting to give advice on standards of professional conduct. As a result, the council formulated a Code of Professional Conduct, its first edition being issued in 1983 and a revised edition, after the receipt of comments from the profession, in 1984.

The aim of this book is to examine some of the theoretical issues surrounding the Code and to explore some of its implications. Theories have been drawn from a wide range of disciplines, moral – philosophy, ethics, psychology, sociology, education and nursing – in order to widen the debate.

Each chapter examines one statement from the Code and explores the concepts and problems that relate to it. We do not suggest that what is discussed is exhaustive of what may be said on each issue, but we hope that the approach will raise some debate, that the book will act as a catalyst.

The breadth of debate is also influenced by the perceptions of the authors which in many ways are very different: male and female, married and single, sociology and psychology, general nursing and psychiatry, Christian and undecided. However, what they have in common is that both are nurses and both are deeply concerned with the standards of care offered to the public and to the development of the profession.

It is hoped that the book will be useful to nurses, midwives and health visitors of all levels and wherever they work. As already indicated, it does not claim to provide definitive answers but to stimulate discussion.

PHILIP BURNARD
CHRISTINE M CHAPMAN
1988

Professional and Ethical Issues

Living languages, like living people, constantly change; they develop, become more sophisticated, sometimes decay and may be abused. The word 'profession' is an example of the dynamic activity affecting words. At one time, to be a member of a profession meant one was either a member of the clergy, a physician or a lawyer: now it frequently means that the occupation so categorised requires either a degree of skill and/or specific knowledge. So we have professional footballers, as well as professional engineers and architects.

In an early attempt to overcome the lack of a succinct definition of the word 'profession', Carr-Saunders and Wilson (1933) stated, 'The term profession ...clearly stands for something. That something is a complex of characteristics.' Unfortunately, this statement does not help a great deal as there is no agreement on what the characteristics are. Most lists of attributes, however, contain the following ideas:

A body of specific knowledge based on research.

For many years nurses were hesitant about claiming a specific body of knowledge. However, if as Hockey (1974) asserts, nursing is a 'unique mix of knowledge and skills, many of which originated in other disciplines', then it may be said that nursing has a body of knowledge. Much of what nurses do has a theoretical basis which is not recognised or made explicit. For example, germ theory lies at the base of all aseptic nursing procedures: whether or not masks or gowns are worn; barrier nursing; lotions used to clean the skin or mouth, and so on. The laws of thermodynamics and other related physical laws underlie procedures such as temperature-taking, tepid sponging and care of the hypothermic patient. Psychological theories have affected views on the visiting of children (and adults) in hospital, the relationship between information, anxiety and pain, talking to the dying patient and helping bereaved relatives. Physiological theories should assist in the way in which medicines are given; assist the patient with elimination; and a great many more activities. Sociological theory contributes to the understanding of the role of the patient and nurse, how organisations function, and patterns of power and other social factors.

The qualifying statement 'based on research' is only gradually becoming true and, as the testing of knowledge increases, there is the exciting discovery that, in many cases, there is more than a 'mix' of knowledge as new knowledge is identified and synthesised.

> The amount and type of knowledge passed on to the new entrants to a profession and the specific skills required are directed by members of that profession and the institutions involved in their eductation are validated by the profession.

This is certainly the case in nursing because the outline curriculum acceptable for registration is controlled by the United Kingdom Central Council and the four National Boards for Nursing, Midwifery and Health Visiting. In addition, the approval of the educational institutions and the qualifying examinations are the responsibilty of the National Boards. Most professionals have their name entered onto a register of licensed practitioners. This register is important in that it informs the public not only that the individual has reached a satisfactory level of competence but that a certain standard of behaviour can be expected. This latter point is exemplified in the next characteristic.

> The attitude of the professional towards the client is one of service on an individual basis, the clients' needs beeing placed before those of the professional.

In that the knowledge and skill possessed by the professional may be relatively difficult for the client to assess, there has to be an element of trust placed by the client in the professional. In turn, the professional must be prepared to accept that trust. In order to reassure the client as to standards of behaviour that can be expected, some professions have an ethical code which underlies their professional conduct. Deviation from this code may result in the professional's name being removed from the register of licenced practitioners.

> Accountability for standards of practice is judged by fellow professionals

and only they are able to make decisions as to whether the quality of service is appropriate.

However, Etzioni (1969) states: 'The ultimate justification of a professional act is that it is, to the best of the professional's knowledge the right act.' This demonstrates the high level of accountability that the professional must have for professional practice.

Public recognition is important to the professional, and the phrase 'he's a real professional' is often used to denote admiration of the skill demonstrated by the individual in a specific sphere of activity. The problem is that many people demonstrate a high level of skill in their job – consider the work of a diamond-cutter or a cabinet-maker – yet these occupations are not normally considered to be professions. The level and type of knowledge underlying the skill and the relationship of the professional with the client are of a different order to that of the tradesman.

Finally,

> Professions tend to develop their own sub-culture.

Greenwood (1957) describes this as 'consciousness of kind' which binds members together. This may be demonstrated by the formation of a professional organisation which not only facilitates this coming together for mutual help and support but, according to Greenwood, allows members to 'Learn and evaluate innovations in theory. This provides a mutually stimulating milieu that is in marked contrast to the milieu of the non-professional.' Such a list does not answer the question: 'When is an occupation a profession?' If an occupation is measured against such a list how many positive 'ticks' are needed for the occupation to be called a profession? How many entitle it to be called a semi-profession? Where is the cut-off point?

As already stated, as far as the 'man in the street' is concerned, it is the certainty of a particular type of behaviour that earns a person the title 'professional' rather than the possession by that occupational group of any number of characteristics. It is for this reason that groups, whether or not recognised as professions, adopt codes of conduct by which their members may be guided. Some codes are very old, an example being the Hippocratic Oath, variants of which are still taken by graduating medical practitioners. Others such as the UKCC's Code of Professional Conduct are relatively new.

What is a Code of Conduct and what is its purpose and standing?

What it is not, is law. This may come as a suprise to many people, especially as in many professions their code of conduct is used to judge professional behaviour and may be cited in disciplinary committees. A code of conduct is what it says it is − a code or guidance regarding appropriate conduct for a specific group of people carrying out specific actions. Many codes of conduct claim to be based on ethical principles (i.e. ICN Code for Nurses 1973); others do not overtly make that claim but nevertheless have ethically-based statements within their pages.

The definition of ethics, like that 'profession', is fraught with difficulty. The *Concise Oxford Dictionary* states that it is the 'science of morals', which raises the question: 'What is meant by morals?' Tschudin (1986) claims that 'ethics is caring', and that 'to act ethically is to care . . . to care for ourselves and others.' This approach is certainly attractive to those who claim to be members of caring professions. However, in a sense this approach is tautological and gives no real, practical guide to action. Indeed, the advocates of euthanasia often justify their claims to the right to end life on the basis that they 'care' and wish to relieve suffering, yet many would question whether such behaviour was indeed ethical. In the place of the word 'ethical' many people would substitute the word 'right' and it is the consideration of actions, beliefs and attitudes that makes up the study of moral philosophy. In an attempt to decide what is 'right', 'good', and 'just', Cambell (1979), trying to separate out the difference between ethics and morals, acknowledged that the Greek and Latin from which the words derive mean more or less the same thing − 'that which is customary or generally accepted' − but then went on to use the word 'morals' to describe the phenomena which are studied by 'ethics'.

The study of ethics may, therefore, be said to have two aspects, the first is related to how people 'should' behave and is based on the age-old debate engaged in by philosophers as to what is good, right and just; and the second aspect, which can almost be considered to be the obverse side of the same coin, is related to what people actually do, and the pressures − personal, cultural, organisational − which influence their actions. The first consideration may lead to statements which ignore the consequences; the second sees the result of action as the most important factor. In making an ethical decision or in drawing up a code of conduct both aspects need to be considered.

Thiroux (1980) has established a set of Principles of Ethics which may be applied to any situation. They are:

–The value of life.
–Goodness or rightness.
–Justice or fairness.
–Truth-telling or honesty.
–Individual freedom.

It is important, according to Thiroux, to consider each of these principles when deciding on action. For example, if it is agreed that life is of supreme value, then when is it appropriate to stop striving to maintain it, i.e. when is death a realistic option? This is the first principle because without it the others are meaningless. However, Thiroux also states: 'Human beings should revere life and accept death', which may help in making a decision to turn off a life-support system. It may also help to remind the nurse that quality of life has to be considered as well as quantity. Yet this fact produces another dilemma; the quality of life enjoyed by a severly handicapped person may appear to be very low indeed to the healthy young observer, yet to the person concerned life may still be precious and worth while.

The question as to the 'goodness' of an action has been debated since Aristotle, with a variety of measures being suggested by which an action may be judged. These range from original intention to the outcome of the activity.

Aristotle (see Chase 1925) claimed that virtue lay in the appropriateness of the object or person for the task, thus a 'good knife' is one that is sharp and cuts cleanly, because cutting is the function of a knife. It may also be aesthetically pleasing to look at or it may be ugly, valuable or of little intrinsic worth, but if it does its job then it is 'good' and produces satisfaction or happiness. At first sight this is an attractive definition and may appear to solve the problem, but closer consideration will reveal some difficulties. What, for example, is the purpose of an individual, and can a person be described as 'good' because that purpose is met? The shorter Scottish Catechism states that 'The chief aim of man is to glorify God and to enjoy Him forever'; while Benjamin Disraeli stated: 'Man . . . is a being born to believe.' Now whether or not you agree with these statements, or prefer to substitute other functions as the purpose for the existence of human life, it is easy to see that there may be individuals, perhaps the physically or mentally handicapped, or aged and infirm, who may be unable to perform the agreed function. Does this fact make them evil? Obviously not. So that while ability to function appropriately may be a useful way of assessing the value of a knife, it is of no help in discussing the value of a person.

Many people would say that everyone knows what is 'right' and 'good' by the way in which his conscience responds, making him feel that something should, or should not, be carried out. This is not a new idea. Bishop Butler in the eighteenth century (1926) developed an elaborate theory of conscience in which he claimed that having and obeying one's conscience was essential to being classified as human. He explained this by comparing the human personality to a watch, whose separate parts are only of use when placed in relationship to each other. Conscience, he claimed, was an essential part of the mechanism of the human personality and without it the individual was incomplete. Further, he claimed that an individual was motivated by three factors. First, by 'particular passions', that is, by basic drives like hunger; some emotional reactions such as fear and anger and 'traits' like shyness or aggression. Secondly, by 'rational calculating principles', which calculate the individual's own long-term happiness, of what Butler called 'cool self-love', and the calculation of the happiness of others, which he described as 'the principle of benevolence'; and thirdly, 'conscience' which would hold the superior position and enable the individual to decide between the rightness of action under the other motivating forces. For an individual to disobey his or her conscience, according to Butler, is to destroy the natural balance of their personality.

All this sounds fine but, of course, people do not always obey their consciences. Another difficulty is that my conscience may say one thing and in an identical situation yours may dictate another. Indeed, it is this very conflict which causes so many problems in nursing/medical practice. One person fully believes that it is wrong to destroy life in any situation and therefore his conscience forbids him to assist in abortions; another believes, equally vehemently, that there are occasions when abortion is appropriate. Both must follow their own conscience and thus no consensus can be reached. Instead, to use Sartre's (1948) words, 'The individual is entirely alone and abandoned in his decision; he, and he alone, must take the responsibilty.' Such a view cannot therefore be the basis of a code of practice to be followed by a group of people, as each must make his own decision.

Another approach taken by a number of people when deciding on a course of action is to consider whether or not they would like it done to themselves. Charles Kingsley (1869) used this principle in his book *The Water Babies* when he developed the character Mrs Do-As-You-Would-Be-Done-By. Kant (1785) too held this point of view but also claimed that morality was doing one's duty for duty's sake. He described a series of actions as 'categorical imperatives' that is to say, they must be followed. These are:

So act that the maxim of your action can become a universal law for all rational beings.

Act as if the maxim of your action were to become by your will a universal law of nature.

So act as to treat humanity, whether in your own person or in that of any other, in every case as an end, never as a mere means.

However, there are problems in applying this law of 'universality' when dealing with people who are themselves different and thus require different consideration. Does a commitment to preserve life mean that every patient who dies must be resuscitated because that is the universal law? Some would argue 'yes', while many would want to say 'it all depends'. Indeed, some would wish the patient to be given the opportunity to request that resuscitation should or should not be carried out, for, if this choice is denied, the patient may be used as a 'means' to enable the nursing or medical staff to comfort themselves with the thought that everything had been done for the patient. Yet Kant said that the person must be an 'end in himself'. Consider the arguments used to support the decision to spend money in one area of health care rather than another – remarks such as 'He is so young' or 'She is old and has had her life': heart transplants before treatment for arthritis, acute care before chronic, and so on. In all these statements 'ends' are implied regarding the worth of individuals in relation to their likely contribution to society: means, not ends in themselves.

More acceptable may be the consideration of whether or not an action produces happiness. The Utilitarians, notably Jeremy Bentham and John Stuart Mill, asserted that what is good is pleasure and happiness, and what is bad is pain. A good action, therefore, is one that produces more pleasure than pain. However, as any parent will know, a child's wishes have often to be denied, thus producing unhappiness, because granting the request may be dangerous for the child. Can such a denial be considered bad? A further problem is that happiness for one group may produce unhappiness for another. Who, then, is to be satisfied? The one with most power? So develops the tyranny of the majority.

From this discussion, it is clear that it is difficult – perhaps impossible – to formulate one rule by which every situation may be judged, so that it can be said with certainty that 'this action is good, right and just'. One common thread running throughout the debate is the conviction that people cannot be treated as a collection of things such as knives, and that each person has to be regarded individually. Indeed, this is one of the first lessons learnt by the new entrant to nursing. All patients must be treated alike.

Even this statement may be contentious: discussion on whether an action is just or fair cannot stop at saying that all must be treated alike when it is quite clear that all are not the same to begin with. Is discrimination, positive or negative, ever justified? We have already considered the problem in relation to expenditure on health care for specific groups. There is an apparent paradox in the statements: 'all people must be treated alike' and 'each person has to be treated as an individual'. This paradox can be easily resolved: the nurse must not differentiate between patients on the grounds of colour, social class, education, attractiveness of personality, and so on; only on the basis of the activity required to meet the patients individual needs. However, this does not help when having to allocate scarce resources.

Schrock (1980) claims that nurses are often less than honest in their dealings with patients, yet honesty and truthfulness make up Thiroux's Fourth Principle. Most people in everyday life support varying degrees of honesty and truth-telling. This is so accepted that the telling of a 'white lie' carries little stigma on the basis that to do so may be kind. Can this ever really be justified? To what extent is the 'whole truth' necessary? Difficult questions, especially when caring for some patients, are nevertheless a principle of morality.

Another aspect of morality relates to the use of equipment and time. Both are easily misappropriated and thus the employer is defrauded. Yet how often is this considered to be stealing?

Finally, comes the principle of individual freedom. This, if present, will influence the way the first four principles are held and acted upon. What is more, it implies autonomy of action so that no one else can be held responsible for the actions of another. Nurses frequently question the extent to which they have autonomy and, therefore, whether they can be held responsible for the care that they give. Codes of conduct assume that the individual is accountable – to what extent are they correct?

What all this apparently leads to is a belief that a moral basis for action has to be rooted in the perception of the intrinsic worth of the individual and that person's right to self-determination. (Christians would back up this respect by explaining that man is created in the image of God.) The debate on what constitutes a person has already been touched upon. Most agree that the definition includes the possession by an individual of human-type characteristics, with a capacity, however small, to communicate and be communicated with (not necessarily by speech). 'Respect of person' in this context requires activity which is a combination of both rational and emotional elements used in a relationship of involvement with other individuals, so that their wishes, thoughts and aspirations are taken into account.

This approach – the respect of persons – has some important implications. First, there is no absolute set of moral rules to guide action, as modification may have to take place in the light of the individual; secondly, the individual is given greater value than society; thirdly, it demmands an attempt to maintain a continuing relationship with the indivdual, so that the person does not become an object to whom things are done. These factors are costly in time, resources and human endeavour and do not provide quick or easy answers.

It is in the light of this type of discussion that the United Kingdom Central Council for Nursing, Midwifery and Health Visiting (UKCC) issued, not a set of rules, but a *Code of Professional Conduct* as guidance for professional practitioners. The first code specifically drawn up for those registered in the United Kingdom was published in 1983. It was circulated to the profession and comments requested. As a result of these comments a revised edition was issued in 1984.

The purpose of the code is summarised in its opening paragraph,

> Each registered nurse, midwife and health visitor shall act, at all times, in such a manner as to justify public trust and confidence, to uphold and enhance the good standing of the profession, to serve the interests of society and above all to safeguard the interests of individual patients and clients.

It is interesting to consider why the UKCC has now produced a Code of Conduct when the International Council of Nurses produced their first code in 1953. The answer lies in the fact that, while nurses in the UK previously used the ICN Code, the 1979 Nurses, Midwives and Health Visitors Act specified for the first time that the functions of the UKCC were to:

> ...establish and improve standards of training and professional conduct . . . and that the powers of the Council shall include that of providing, in such a manner as it thinks fit, advice for nurses,

midwives and health visitors on standards of professional conduct.

The provision of the code has not been welcomed by all. This is partly due to a misunderstanding of its function, fear that it might become a stick with which to beat the profession, and concern that it may be unrealistic in its demands. Certainly a great deal of the concern expressed has been due to some of the guidance not being understood and the UKCC has attempted to increase understanding of some specific issues by the publication of explanatory leaflets.

Rumbold (1986) claims that professional codes serve three main functions:

1. To reasure the public.
2. To provide guidlines for the profession to regulate and discipline its members.
3. To provide a framework on which individual members can formulate decisions.

It is to explore these issues that this book has been written.

REFERENCES

Butler, J. (1726) Sermons on Human Nature. In *Fifteen Sermons*. Roberts, T.A. (ed.) (1970) SPCK: London.

Cambell, A.V. (1979) Plato. Apology 3A. In *Moral Dilemmas in Medicine*. Churchill Livingstone: Edinburgh.

Carr-Saunders, A.M. & Wilson, P.A. (1964) *The Professions*. F. Cass: London.

Chapman, C.M. (1976) The use of Sociological Theories and Models in Nursing. *Journal of Advanced Nursing* 1:111-127.

Chase, D.P. (trans. 1925) Aristotle, *Nichomachean Ethics*. Dent: London.

Etzioni, A. (ed.) (1969) *The Semi-Professions and Their Organization*. Free Press: New York.

Greenwood, E. (1957) Attributes of a Profession. In *Social Work* **II**,3, 45-55. National Association of Social Workers, Washington.

Hockey, L. (1974) *Forschung im Bereich der Pflege*. Paper presented to Fortbildungskongress für psychiatrisches Krankenpflegepersonal und Sozialarbeite, Heidelberg October 1973. Osterreichische Krankenpflege Zeitschrift 27,2, pp. 41-48.

International Council of Nurses (1973) *Code for Nurses*. ICN: Geneva.

Kant, I. (1785) *Fundamental Principles of the Metaphysics of Morals* (trans. Abbott. T.K.). Library of Literal Arts: New York.

Kingsley, C.C. (1885) *The Water Babies*. Garland: London (1976).

Mills, J.S. (1869) *Utilitarianism*. Longmans: London.

Nurses, Midwives and Health Visitors Act 1979. HMSO London.

Rumbold, G. (1986) *Ethics in Nursing Practice*: Baillière Tindall: London

Sartre, J.P. (1984) *Existentialism and Humanism*. Methuen: London.

Schrock. R. (1980) A Question of Honesty in Nursing Practice. *Journal of Advanced Nursing.* **5,**2, 135-148.

Thiroux, J.P. (1980) *Ethics, Theory and Practice* (2nd ed.) Glencoe Publishing Company Inc. Cal.

Tschudin, V. (1986) *Ethics in Nursing: The Caring Relationship.* Heinemann Nursing: London.

United Kingdom Central Council (1983 and 1984) *Code of Professional Conduct.*

CHAPTER 1

Promoting and Safeguarding the Interests of Patients

Act always in such a way as to promote and safeguard the
well-being and interests of patients/clients.

Much time and energy has been devoted to discussing the question
'What is nursing?' The answer is complicated by the fact that nurses
are not a homogeneous group of people, all engaged in virtually
identical tasks. On the contrary, nurses can be found in almost all
walks of life: caring for infants and the aged; working in operating
theatres and factories; in the midst of the battle field and giving aid
in famine-stricken lands; providing highly technical care and
teaching healthy living. So all-encompassing is the role of the nurse
that it is tempting to answer the question 'What is nursing' by saying
that it is 'what nurses do.' However, such an answer evades the
purpose to the question which is to decide what, if anything, can be
identified as the essential nature of the profession.

To answer the question then, it is important to consider not only the
tasks performed by nurses but the motivation underlying the tasks.
One factor that is clear is that no matter where nurses work or what
the nature of the task may be, nursing involves a personal
interaction between one individual, the nurse, and another
individual, the patient or client. That is not to ignore the fact that
sometimes the nurse is involved with a group of patients or that any
indivdual nurse may be part of a health care team; nevertheless, at
the point of contact it is individual with individual. Henderson
(1956) defined nursing as:

> . . . primarily assisting the individual (sick or well) in the performance
> of those activities contributing to health, or its recovery (or to a

peaceful death) that he would perform unaided if he had the necessary strength, will or knowledge. It is likewise the unique contribution of nursing to help the individual to be independent of such assistance as soon as possible.

Florence Nightingale (1859) was not happy with the word 'nursing'. She said that she used it for the want of another! However, she described the work done by nurses as 'designed to keep people well, to help them to avoid disease, and to restore them to their highest level of health'.

What both these definitions have in common is that they focus on the individual patient or client, they stress the maintenance of health and the prevention of disease, and they emphasise the aim of patient independence. The roles of nurse and patient/client are complementary. Without the presence of a patient/client there would be no need of a nurse. (The word nurse in this context is used in its generic sense and therefore includes all branches of care provided by nurses.)

How does a person become a patient? Sociologists argue that this occurs in a variety of ways. Talcott Parsons (1966) suggests that a person has only the right to be called 'sick' if that person seeks competent help, actively desires to get well and co-operates in the activity designed to assist in the return to health. In this case the individual is excused other roles. Certainly, this is the way society works, in that it demands certification by a medical practitioner if the indisposition lasts for more than a few days.

Robinson (1971), however, showed in his study of families in Swansea that the presence of physical symptoms was not always sufficient to ensure that a person sought medical advice. Frequently, the difficulty of being excused social roles, the danger of losing a job if 'off sick', the problem of finding someone to care for children, and other non-medical social factors, often meant that the person deferred or sacrificed the right to be classified as sick and failed to seek help.

It is always difficult to be certain why any person enters nursing but when asked, almost all say something to the effect that they want to help and care for people. Certainly, that is the image that the public has of a nurse – 'one who cares'. What is more, they expect that this care will be of a personal nature, that is, the nurse will care for them not just as a 'patient' but as an individual. Jourard (1971) put it like this: 'One of the events which we believe inspires hope in a patient is the conviction that someone cares about him.' If this is true then the nature of the nurse/patient relationship is of prime importance.

The problem is that most nurses find themselves working in an organisation which may have other aims than that of fostering effective interpersonal relationships, and this is true even of those who work outside traditional health care institutions. Melia (1981) found that most nurses were concerned with 'getting the work done' and it is often the case that qualified nurses are rewarded for bureaucratic efficiency rather than for the quality of the care they provide. This is in stark contrast to the first guidance given in the Code which enjoins the nurse to 'Act always in such a way as to promote and safeguard the well-being and interests of patients/clients.'

To be able to assess what are the interests of the patient or client the nurse has to have time to develop an interpersonal relationship and to foster a feeling of empathy. The development of empathy requires the nurse to 'step into the shoes' of the patient in order to perceive the world through his eyes and to feel what he feels. Armed with this knowledge the nurse has then to return to the role of a nurse using the knowledge gained to enhance the care given. This does require that the nurse becomes involved with the patient, an activity frequently frowned on in the past and still regarded with suspicion by many as being 'unprofessional'. What is unprofessional is an impersonal approach which results in all patients being treated as if they are identical, which is clearly not the case.

To return to Jourard (1964):

> Much of contemporary interpersonal competence seems to entail success in getting patients to conform to the roles they are supposed to play in the social system of the hospital so that the system will work smoothly, work will get done faster and the patients will be less of a bother to care for.

What an indictment of a group of people who apparently entered the profession to care for others!

The problem is that in some cases the nurse's desire to give physical care is such that the patient is not allowed to 'return to independence' even though that is an important aspect of care. Talcott Parsons, in defining the role of the patient, said that not only must the person seek competent help and positively wish to recover but he also emphasised that the patient must comply with the treatment offered. This may be appropriate, but all care-givers need to remember that, in the final analysis the individual is responsible for his own life unless, as described by Henderson (1966), they do not have the strength, knowledge or will.

All health care professionals have problems in acknowledging that the patient/client may not wish to accept the advice that they are given. There is always the assumption that the doctor or nurse knows best yet, as the title of a famous play says, 'Whose life is it anyway?'

Another important aspect of the role of the nurse in acting always in the best interest of the patient/client is that of health educator. It is often felt that this is an aspect of care which is the sole responsibility of those specially trained for the task, such as the health visitor or occupational health nurse. Nothing could be further from the truth: nurses, by virtue of the respect with which they are held, and the fact that they are frequently in close contact with individuals and their families, are in a superb position not only to become involved in teaching healthy living but also by their example may demonstrate such living in practice. This is an awesome responsibility and should make any nurse who is obese, or who smokes, or who indulges in any other questionable life-style, stop and consider that by such actions the best interests of the patient or client may not be served. It may be argued that just as patients/clients have the right to self-determination in regard to their own life, so the nurse has equal rights. In one sense this is true but, as already argued in the Introduction, by belonging to a profession the nurse assumes certain responsibilities and in return is accorded special rights. Indeed, rights and duties can be seen as the opposite sides of the same coin.

What is meant by the words 'right' and 'duty'? Benn and Peters (1959) argue that a right and a duty are different terms for the same normative relationship (i.e. situation based on rules), varying according to the position from which the situation is regarded: in other words, one person's rights become another person's duties. Rights also imply duties in another sense, in that the enjoyment by an individual of specific rights is usually conditional on the performance by that individual of specific duties.

What then are the rights and responsibilities of nurses and patients when involved in patient care? The activity of nursing has undergone revision in the last twenty years: no longer is it seen as a collection of tasks performed on a passive patient but as a partnership between the nurse and the patient where both endeavour to achieve agreed health care goals. This implies an activity involving assessment, goal-setting, planned intervention and evaluation of progress. All this is dependent on effective communication and interaction, although, as already discussed, the nurse may have to act where the patient does not have the strength, knowledge or will to act for him or herself.

The ICN Code for Nurses denotes four main areas of responsibility for the nurse: to promote health, to prevent illness, to restore health and to alleviate suffering. Continuing the idea that one person's rights are another person's duties a picture emerges as shown in Table 1.1.

Nurses' Duties	Patients' Rights
To promote health	Health or
To prevent illness	a
To restore health	peaceful
To alleviate suffering	death.

Figure 1.1

Stockwell (1972) also found that patients felt that they had the right to receive:

- Skilled care – 'a nurse you can depend on'.
- Attention to 'trivial matters'.
- More information.
- More opportunity to voice worries and needs.

One of the responsibilities of the nurse is to act as the patient's advocate in situations where the patient is unable to act for himself. Advocacy is often a misunderstood concept – the *Concise Oxford Dictionary* defines an advocate as being '...one who pleads or speaks for another.' Patients frequently find it difficult to express fully their needs and fears. The nurse who has truly cultivated the skill of empathy and who is in frequent personal interaction with the patient may be able to interpret the patient's needs to others and to act as a go-between when other health care professionals appear, to the patient, to be unapproachable. This may also require the nurse to explain to the patient possible alternative lines of treatment and to ensure that he is fully aware of the implications before consent to treatment is given. This does not absolve other health care professionals from their responsibility to act in the best interest of the patient, and most will do so, but it does place the nurse, who has this close, continuing relationship with the patient, in a special position of responsibility. Brown (1985) claims that 'advocacy is a means of transferring power back to the patient'.

Figure 1.2 Rights and Responsibilities of the Nurse and Patient

	NURSE		PATIENT	
Rights	Responsibilities	Rights	Responsibilities
To have:	*To give:*	*To receive:*	*To:*
experience	skilled care	skilled care	co-operate
recognition	individual care	individual care	conform to routine
reward	information	information	
status money gratitude	emotional support	empathy	be grateful

In summary, Styles (1983) in *Declaration of Belief About the Nature and Purpose of Nursing* says in Item 4:

I believe in nursing as a humanistic field in which the fullness, self-respect, self-determination, and humanity of the nurse engage the fullness, self-respect, self-determination, and the humanity of the client.

This is surely acting in the best interests of the patient/client.

REFERENCES

Benn S.I. and Peters R.S. (1959) *Social Principles and the Democratic State.* Allen and Unwin: London.

Brown M. (1985) Matter of Commitment. *Nursing Times,* **81 (18)**, 26-27.

Henderson. V. (1966) *Basic Principles of Nursing Care.* International Council of Nurses: Geneva.

ICN (1973) *Code for Nurses.* International Council for Nurses: Switzerland.

Jourard. S.M. (1964) *The Transparent Self.* Van Nostrand: New York.

Jourard. S.M. (1971) *The Transparent Self.* Van Nostrand: New York.

Melia, K.M. (1981) Student nurses' accounts of their work and training: a qualitative analysis. Unpublished PhD Thesis, University of Edinburgh.

Nightingale. F. (1859) *Notes on Nursing.* (reprinted 1970). Dent: London

Parsons, T. (1966) On becoming a patient. In *A Sociological Framework for Patient Care,* eds. Folta J.R. and Deck E.S. John Wiley and Sons: Chichester.

Robinson, D. (1971) *The Process of Becoming Ill.* Routledge & Kegan Paul: London.

Stockwell F. (1972) *The Unpopular Patient.* Royal College of Nursing: London.

Styles. M. (1983) *Nursing: Towards a New Endowment.* Mosby: St Louis.

CHAPTER 2

Responsibility in Action

Ensure that no action or omission on his/her part or within his/her sphere of influence is detrimental to the condition or safety of patients/clients.

The second article in the Code of Professional Conduct emphasises both the positive action and the negative omission side of the nurse's role, and also points out that it may not be the nurse's direct activity that is under consideration but also the action of others within the sphere of influence.

> The ultimate justification of a professional act is that it is, to the best of the professional's knowledge, the right act. (Etzioni 1969)

Implicit in this quotation is the idea that the professional will take responsibility for the action because it is, in the specific circumstances, 'right'. We have already discussed the way in which the goodness or rightness of an action can be judged; the focus of this chapter shifts to the burden of responsibility or, to adopt the term most frequently used these days, 'accountability'.

The words 'accountability' and 'responsibility' are frequently used synonymously: however, there is a difference. While people may be held to be responsible for an action they may not always be asked to 'account' for it. The nurse, however, is not only responsible for the care given but should be able to explain why it was given in the way it is. It is necessary for the nurse not only to be concerned with the outcome of the action but she must understand its origins and the process of carrying it out. For example, a nurse may be responsible for getting a patient out of bed 12 hours after major surgery; however to be held accountable for this action implies that she has a reason for this move other than just that 'Sister said so' and that the possible outcomes are understood. This means that the accountable nurse will understand both the dangers of immobility and the incidence of deep vein thrombosis, but also the possible unacceptable fall in blood pressure that may occur, thus increasing the risk of shock. Understanding both possible consequences of getting the patient out of bed she will make a decision as to the best course of action for that specific patient which may not be the same decision for the patient in the next bed.

It is quite clear, therefore, that to be accountable requires knowledge so that the relative benefits or otherwise of alternative forms of action can be assessed. This means that while a student may be held responsible for care given to the patient it is frequently not possible for the learner to be held accountable: she may not yet have the academic knowledge or the practical experience to assess fully the situation prior to carrying out the care. This has major implications in the use of the nursing process in that assessment of the individual patient is fundamental to all planning of nursing care. While it may be possible for a student to obtain and record information from the patient, the significance of the data, the identification of the nursing problems and the planning of care may have to be left to, or be supervised by, the qualified nurse.

However it is not as simple as that. Knowledge should be research-based and up-to-date if it is to be 'the best', and this has implications for continuing education as a basis for accountability in practice. The requirement for the nurse to re-register every three years with evidence of the maintenance of professional knowledge is an attempt to ensure that all patients receive the highest level of care and that the qualified nurse can really be seen to be in a position of accountability.

To be accountable also requires authority. It is of little value if the nurse knows what is the most appropriate method of care if some other person or circumstance prevents that care being given. Bureaucratic organisations often reject the idea of individual authority by insisting on 'chains of command', adherence to rules and policies, with no flexibility or discretion allowed to the individual practitioner. While it is easy to understand how managers, in assuming ultimate accountability for the total organisation, feel they need the protection of such rules they are obviously less suitable in the health care setting, where each client/patient interaction is different, than in a factory that produces identical goods.

To summarise, therefore: to be accountable the nurse requires not only the appropriate up-to-date research-based knowledge, but also the authority to act with a reasonable degree of autonomy. It is a waste of resources and a negation of expectations to prepare a nurse for three or more years to act in accordance with knowledge and to draw on experience gained in the clinical situation if individual judgement is then denied by either managerial style and/or tradition.

There are, of course, areas of potential conflict between either fellow nurses whose professional judgement may advocate alternative forms of action or, possibly, between the nurses and members of other professions, and these situations are discussed later. In addition, there may be conflict with the patient who has different expectations of what is appropriate care. This requires effective nurse/patient communication so that the patient understands the reason for the proposed action and the nurse understands the patient's point of view. However, it is important to appreciate that in the end the patient has the final right to decide the care to be given or not given. In this case, the nurse may have to surrender to the autonomy of the patient who then assumes accountability for the decision. Nurses, therefore, are primarily accountable to their patients and then to their colleagues, the profession and the public.

When discussing accountability the emphasis is generally placed on 'doing'; however, it is equally important to appreciate that accountability also extends to 'not doing' and that the omission of appropriate care is as serious as the performance of inappropriate care.

There is little doubt that for a nurse to fail to give a drug is a serious failure of care. Such an omission may prejudice the patient's chance of recovery, result in prolonged pain, or lead to the development of organisms that are resistant to the drug. Equally negligent is the failure to record that the drug has been given as this may result in its being given again in too short a time interval.

Health visitors often feel that their actions are less open to abuse than those of nurses engaged in clinical practice. However, failure to carry out developmental tests on children or to record the results of such tests may prejudice the growth and development of a child.

At managerial level the failure to check that delegated responsibilities have been met may also be counted as negligence, as may not ensuring that nurses have sufficient resources to carry out such tasks.

One specific act of omission that may occur is that caused by industrial action. Members of the Royal College of Nursing have rejected on many occasions the deletion of Rule 12 in the constitution which forbids such action, as they appreciate that it is not possible in the context of patient care. However, in 1979 industrial action was taken by nurses belonging to other trade unions and as a result the then statutory body the General Nursing Council for England and Wales issued the following statement:

> The Council is of the opinion that if a nurse puts the health, safety or welfare of his or her patients at risk by taking strike or other industrial action he or she would have a case to answer on the score of professional misconduct, just as he or she would if the health, safety or welfare of patients were put at risk by any other action on his or her part.

Subsequent to this statement, two charge nurses working in a Northern Ireland psychiatric hospital were found guilty of misconduct by the GNC for 'absenting themselves from duty without good reason', during a strike called by the Confederation of Health Service Employees. During the case the Chairman of the committee asked the members to consider the following questions: 'Have the actions of the respondent damaged the public confidence in the profession as a whole?' and: 'Have the actions resulted in actual or potential harm to any member of the vunerable public?'.

On the evidence it was stated that one of the charge nurses was reluctant to strike but feared being labelled as a 'blackleg'. While it is possible to understand that fear, especially when related to a comparatively closed community such as a psychiatric hospital, it is obvious that the chief concern of the nurse must be the safety of the patients in his/her care.

At the time the debate on the 'right to strike' was hotly pursued. Trades unions other than the RCN called the GNC's statement a threat, intimidation and blackmail. The then Registrar of the GNC replied in an article published in the *Nursing Mirror* (Storey, 1979) in the following terms:

> The statement is not about taking industrial action, it is not about the nurses' right to strike, it is not about trades union activity,

management/staff relationships, resource allocation or the many other issues which have arisen as a result of misinterpretation. It is about the health, safety and welfare of patients and the particular responsibility the qualified nurse holds in not placing the patient(s) at risk.

She also referred readers to the ACAS Code of Practice under the heading 'Responsibilities – Individual Employee' which states:

Some employees have special obligations arising from membership of a profession and are liable to incur penalties if they disregard them. These may include, for example, in regard to health safety and welfare, over and above those which are shared by the Community as a whole.

A professional employee who belongs to a trades union should respect the obligations he has voluntarily taken on by joining the union, BUT he should not, when acting in his professional capacity, be called upon by his trade union to take action which would conflict with the standards of work or conduct laid down by his profession if that action would endanger:

1. Public health or safety,
2. The health of an individual needing medical care or other treatment,
3. The well-being of an individual needing care through the personal social services.

Such statements are clear and unambiguous and while sympathy must be felt for nurses who are frustrated in their endeavours to obtain action from either their employers or the government, it is obvious that consideration of the patient/client must come first.

It is important to consider when an action or omission may be considered to be a mistake based on professional misjudgement and when such action or omission is negligence. Brazier (1987) explains that:

A nurse will be judged in accordance with the standard of skill and carefulness to be expected of a nurse in this position and speciality and with this seniority. A midwife must show a midwife's skill. It is not enough, for example, to display only the standard of an SRN who has done thirteen weeks' obstetrics. A midwife holds herself out as a specialist. . . . the more independent the nurse's function, the greater the risk of finding liability.

Although this last statement refers to midwives, nurses are also accountable and therefore may find themselves liable for negligence if they fail to follow instructions given them by a physician or if they deviate from health authority policy. In some instances the negligence may shared, as in the cases where, while the nurse has not met the appropriate standard of care, management may also be at fault by not ensuring that resources and policies make the achievement of that standard possible.

The sphere of influence of the nurse is considerable. Not only does it encompass those with whom she has an explicit or implicit contract to provide care but also those who may ask for help and advice informally. Thus, while the patient on the ward has, to all intents and purposes, entered into a contract-like relationship with the nurse, the neighbour who seeks advice over the garden fence also has the right to expect skilled professional information. True, the nurse is not contracted to provide such information or help, but once the role is accepted then there is a duty to ensure that it is completed in an appropriate manner. The nurse remains a nurse when practising nursing whether on or off duty, whether acting in a voluntary capacity or as a paid professional: accountability for action is inescapable.

The accountability of those who teach nurses must, in the first instance, be to their students, although indirectly they are also accountable to patients and clients, for if the material they teach is inaccurate or out-of-date then the student may unwittingly give inappropriate or even dangerous care.

This prime accountability to students may bring the teacher into conflict with nurses in managerial positions who quite properly are accountable for providing an adequate supply of manpower to wards and other areas of care. The conflict arises in times of staff shortage when the manager may wish to utilise a student in her employee role to fill a need for a 'pair of hands' while the teacher may see that the student's educational needs require experience in a totally different clinical area.

Managers of care may find themselves in other situations where it may be difficult to decide with whom accountability lies. Bureaucratic institutions have many goals and while it is probable that all who are employed in the Health Service have as a prime goal the welfare of their patients and clients there are also the goals of efficiency and cost-effectiveness to be considered. In addition, as spenders of the money contributed in taxes by the whole community there is a sense in which the manager has accountability to the population at large. The balance that has to be maintained between these sometimes conflicting areas of responsibility is a difficult one. The danger is that the loudest voice will be the one that is heeded and that in some cases the groups that need care the most will be the ones most neglected. Nurses in managerial positions therefore have to be very clear about their sphere of accountability, providing resources to enable others to fulfill their role of giving care while also being responsible for the expenditure of money.

Professional accountability is frequently a complex issue: nevertheless, it is not one that can be put to one side. Once a member of the profession, the nurse cannot escape this burden no matter what role she plays.

REFERENCES

Brazier M. (1987) *Medicine, Patients and the Law.* Penguin Books: Harmondsworth.
Etzioni A. (1969) *The Semi-professions and their Organisation.* Free Press: New York.
Storey M. (1979) Editorial, *Nursing Mirror* 4 October.

CHAPTER 3

Professional Knowledge and Competence

*Take every reasonable opportunity to maintain and improve
professional knowledge and competence.*

At the moment, basic nurse education is a type of apprenticeship. That is to say, student nurses work in the clinical situation and take time away for periods of study. Now at first sight this may seem to be a reasonable state of affairs: student nurses gain practical experience alongside the theoretical inputs from the school of nursing. In practice, the situation is different. Schools of nursing can become remote from clinical practice and staff working in the clinical situation (because of their own distance from training) come to view the school of nursing as idealistic or out of touch with reality. Nor is there evidence that the posts of clinical teacher or joint appointees (tutors with part-responsibility as charge nurses) make any difference to this division between school and clinical area. Project 2000 (UKCC 1986) may change much of this but it is worth considering why such problems have arisen.

One important reason for the theory/practice divide may be the fact of nurse education's adherence to a 'front-end' model of education (Jarvis 1983a); that is to say, that the three years' training that leads to registration as a nurse currently comes all together at the beginning of the nurse's career. Figure 3.1 illustrates this diagrammatically.

Within this model, the nurse is deemed to be competent to enter the profession fully, after the basic three years, and at the present is not required to undertake any educational course following that first three years, in order to continue to practise. It is notable that, at the time of writing, the UKCC is considering introducing compulsory 'refresher' courses for all trained nurses. At present, many nurses *do* choose to pursue other educational courses and a wide range of such courses exist, ranging from two- to three-day workshops to

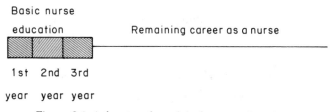

Figure 3.1 A front-end model of nurse education

Master of Nursing programmes. The fact remains, however, that at present there is no *obligation* for the nurse to continue education after the first three years. (Most hospitals have a tutor with special responsibility for postbasic and continuing education but their task is a difficult one given the lack of obligation in the legal sense.)

There is, however, a *moral* obligation for the nurse to continue education. Alfred North Whitehead, the philosopher of science, noted that 'Knowledge keeps no better than fish!' (Whitehead 1932). Knowledge soon becomes 'dead' knowledge – knowledge that is no longer relevant or accurate. The same can be said of skills. The skills learnt during basic nurse education are hardly likely to be sufficient throughout a nursing career. If the nurse is to remain a safe practitioner, knowledge and skills must be kept up-to-date.

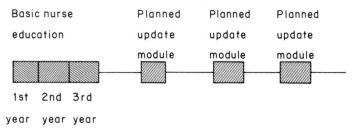

Figure 3.2 A continuing education model of nurse education.

In order to consider this updating process, it may be useful to look at alternatives to the front-end model of education. Figure 3.2 illustrates the continuing education model. In this model the three-year basic education course is retained and planned modules are introduced at, say, yearly intervals. In this way, nurses continue the process of education throughout their careers. The objection may be made here that this model is the one already offered by all hospitals that employ a postbasic or continuing education tutor? In reality, this is not the case. Postbasic education for nurses is rarely *systematically* organised in order that *all* nurses should benefit from regular up-dating.

This model can be adopted by the individual nurse. Every nurse can, if she wishes, regularly review her own level of knowledge and skills and undertake to enroll on a postbasic course in order to make good any deficit. As we shall see, however, there are other ways of tackling the problem. Two obvious drawbacks to this approach may be noted. First, just because the individual nurse identifies particular learning needs does not mean that her desire to undertake a further course of study will necessarily be supported by her manager. Indeed, until further education for nurses becomes mandatory it seems likely that many nurses will *not* find support for their further education. Secondly, the approach may be a haphazard one. It may be relatively easy to review knowledge and skills when we feel highly motivated – it is not so easy after we have been qualified for a few years, and it possibly gets more difficult as we get older.

Educational activities

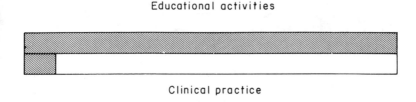

Clinical practice

Nursing career

Figure 3.3 A lifelong education model of nurse education

Figure 3.3 offers a second alternative,that of lifelong education. In this model, following a very short educational input to orient the nurse within the profession, education itself is seen as a major part of the nurse's career, throughout that career. The lifelong education model acknowledges that *all* knowledge is ephemeral and subject to revision and must be modified in the light of research, personal experience, and conceptual and theoretical changes. Skills are also viewed as *evolving* throughout the nurse's career. We do not learn a set of skills which last throughout a working life but modify our skills, as we do our knowledge, through the light of professional and educational developments. Lifelong education is as much a *philosophy* or approach to education as it is a curriculum plan.

Lifelong education as a philosophy may be used for decision-making in nurse education after further consideration about the nature of education itself. In order to make such a decision clearer, two ideal models of the curriculum are offered. An ideal model is one that sets out an example of the sorts of thing that typify one approach. By curriculum is meant all those activities that go to make

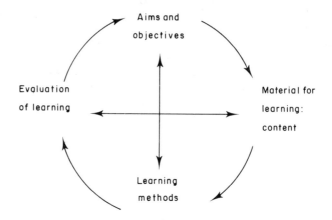

Figure 3.4 A curriculum model

up the educational process: the setting of aims and objectives, the selection of materials for learning, methods of learning and evaluation methods. A typical curriculum model is illustrated in Figure 3.4. In this model, all aspects of the model relate to each other, and the educational process is continuous. Education, then, is not something received once and for all but is a continuous, dynamic process of intellectual growth and development.

Two ideal models of the curriculum can now be described by reference to Figure 3.5. The two models are known as the 'classical' and the 'romantic'. These terms have been used by a variety of writers, including the novelist, Robert Pirsig (1976) and the educationalist, Dennis Lawton (1973), who uses them to make comparisons between types of curricula in a similar way to the comparisons made here.

	Classical Curriculum	Romantic Curriculum
Basic focus of the educational process	Teacher-centred	Student-centred
Aim of the educational process	Teaching	Learning
Aims and objectives	Set by the teacher	Negotiated by teacher with learners
Materials for learning: contents	Decided by teacher	Evolved out of the relationship between teacher and learner
Learner methods	Predetermined by teacher	Decided upon by teacher and learner
Evaluation	Examinations set by teacher	Self and peer evaluation
Nature of knowledge concepts	Absolutist: 'facts exist	Relative knowledge is dependent upon the one who knows
Similar education concepts	'Banking' approach to education (Freire) pedagogy (Knowles)	'Problem-posing approach' (Freire) andragogy (Knowles)

Figure 3.5 Two ideal models of the curriculum

It is asserted that the two curriculum models offer two very different views of the nature of education, and a closer examination of the differences between them may help to illustrate this. The classical model is teacher-centred and its aims is teaching – that is to say, the teacher is perhaps a more important figure than the student. The teacher is seen as the 'one who knows' and the student as the 'one who comes to learn'. The romantic model is student-centred and its main aim is learning. Here, the teacher acts as a 'facilitator of learning' (Rogers 1983). A facilitator is *not* a teacher but one who helps others to learn for themselves. A parallel may be drawn between the traditional nurse who 'cared' for the patient (who was a passive recipient of that care) and the 'modern' nurse who is concerned with enabling the patient to care for himself. So it is in education: in the classical model, the teacher teaches: in the romantic model, the teacher facilitates learning.

Many things follow from this basic difference. In the classical model, aims and objectives are predetermined by the teacher. Lessons are pre-planned independently of the students and the teacher draws up the overall timetable. In the romantic model, aims and objectives are negotiated with the students: student needs and wants are identified, and lessons and the timetable are built around them. So it is with learning methods. In the classical model teaching methods are determined by the teacher. In the romantic model they are chosen through collaboration with the students in order that the students' needs are most suitably met. Evaluation in the classical model is by tests and examinations, set by the teacher. The teacher, having taught, wishes to find out if the learners have learned! In the romantic model both teacher and students engage in self- and peer-evaluation (Kilty 1981: Burnard 1987) wherby each learner (and the teacher) assesses her own performance throughout a 'block' or term and then receives feedback on her performance from her colleagues.

It will be seen that the classical model involves 'teaching from above' whilst the romantic model involves the 'education of equals' (Jarvis 1983b). In the romantic model both teacher and students are 'fellow travellers', for, as we see from Figure 3.5, the view of knowledge is relative. Knowledge is something that grows out of the information and experience that is personal to each individual. Because each person views the world differently from other people, so individual 'knowledge' of the world will be different. In the classical model, knowledge is not relative: there are 'facts' out there in the world that are discernible. It is the teacher's task to pass on those facts. Thus, in the classical model, knowledge is 'impartial' and is unchanged by the one who knows it (Peters 1969).

A distinction similar to the classical/romantic comparison is made by Paulo Freire (1970) when he describes the 'banking' concept of education versus the 'problem-posing' concept. The banking concept involves the teacher filling the students with information which is then 'cashed-out' during examinations. In this model 'more' knowledge is virtually equivalent to 'better-educated'. Alternatively, the problem-posing approach is a means of education through dialogue. Teacher and student meet and exchange ideas through a heated, critical debate − neither teacher nor student has the 'right' answer: there is room for a variety of possibilities.

Malcolm Knowles, the American educator, has used the term *andragogy* to describe negotiated adult education as opposed to *pedagogy* or prescribed child education (Knowles 1981). Knowles argues that negotiated learning is that most appropriate for adults because of (a) the wealth of personal experience that they bring to the learning situation, (b) the fragile nature of their self-concept, and (c) their need to *use* what they learn in a practical sense. As nurses *begin* their training at 18 years of age, it is clear that all nurses *begin* as adults and therefore Knowles' concept of andragogy may have much value in nurse education (Burnard 1985a). It is certainly possible to argue that traditional nurse education has tended to be of the classical, banking type and as modern nursing's aim is to produce the more autonomous patient it would seem reasonable to argue for an educational system that gave nurse learners more control over their educational process. It seems difficult to see how autonomy in nursing can be encouraged unless there is also a degree of learner autonomy in nurse education.

Returning to the concept of lifelong education, it may be seen that the 'romantic' approach to education may be the most appropriate model for fostering such a development. Romantic educational practices involve negotiation, attention to personal needs and wants. They also place much of the *responsibility* for learning firmly with the learner. Indeed, Rogers (1983) argues that it is not impossible to teach anyone anything: they can only be helped to learn. Thus, personal responsibility in the learning process is not only advisable but an essential component. An appreciation of the romantic curriculum can enable nurse tutors, students and clinical practitioners to prepare themselves for lifelong learning.

On the other hand, there is also a clear place for the 'classical' approach. Whilst it has been argued here that the two approaches begin from different theoretical positions, there is no reason why both classical and romantic approaches cannot be used. There are aspects of the nursing curriculum which need to be 'taught', in the sense of passing on of concrete knowledge and skills. All nurses need a sound knowledge and skills base from which to work and there may be sound economic reasons why, in the initial stages of nurse education, the 'classical' approach can be useful. If nurses are 'taught' certain basic approaches to learning, ways of developing theories, methods of using learning resources (books, articles, videos, libraries, bibliographies, etc.), they may later move on to a more 'romantic' approach, where they can use those basic learning skills efficiently and effectively.

The suggestion here is that learners begin from the classical approach to the curriculum and move towards the romantic approach as a means of working within the lifelong education model (Figure 3.6). In this way, there is a move from initial dependence on tutorial staff to an increasing state of independence and self-motivation. Linked to this educational process is the fact of clinical experience. As we have seen in the lifelong learning model, both educational and clinical processes go hand in hand. A valuable method of ensuring that they do is through the use of experiential learning.

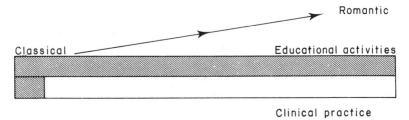

Figure 3.6 Linking lifelong education with the classical/romantic curriculum

Experiential learning is learning through direct experience. It is 'personal' learning and, as such, has much in common with the concepts contained within the idea of the romantic curriculum. Experiential learning is most often linked with the learning of interpersonal skills – listening, counselling, talking to others, managing other people's distress, and so forth (Heron 1973; Burnard 1985b; Kagan 1986). It does, however, also have much wider application. The experiential learning cycle (Figure 3.7) can be used to 'process' *any* practical experience.

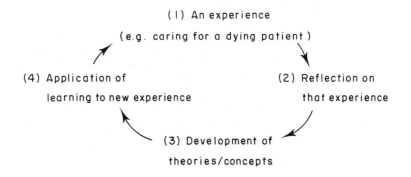

Figure 3.7 The experiential learning cycle

The experiential learning cycle has four stages. Stage 1 is the experience itself (caring for a dying patient, talking to relatives, working in theatre, and so forth). Stage 2 involves the process of quietly reflecting on that experience and attempting to recall all or most aspects of it, good and bad. This reflective period is, perhaps, the most important stage in the cycle. It is tempting to think that a person *always* learns from experience: the fact is, perhaps, that a person *only* learns from experience if that experience is reflected upon. Experience that just 'happens' is rarely of any lasting value, it goes by unnoticed and unremarked.

In Stage 3 of the cycle, new learning in the form of theories and concepts is drawn out of the experience. Here, then, once the reflective period has taken place, the individual 'makes sense' of his experience and relates it to past experience and to the literature and research on the topic. Again, this period of 'making sense' is very important. It is insufficient merely to acknowledge that an experience has occurred; the full implications of that experience need to be explored if new learning is to take place. In Stage 4, that new learning is applied in practice. In the context of nursing, this application will usually be in the clinical situation. Figure 3.8 offers an example of the experiential learning cycle in use.

Stage One: An Experience: Caring for a Dying Patient

Stage Two: Reflection on that Experience
        personal involvement/emotion
        consideration of patient's physical needs
        difficulty in *talking* to patient
        patient's spiritual needs?
        patient's knowledge about their own predicament
        my knowledge of the patient
        my *own* thoughts about dying
        my relationship with other staff
        pain management, etc.

Stage Three: Development of Theories/Concepts
        need for *personal* interpersonal skills training
        stages of dying? Kubler-Ross?
        facing death and spiritual needs: is there a direct
        relationship? Check literature, etc.

Stage Four: Application of Learning to New Experience
        caring, more sensitively, more knowledgeably

Figure 3.8 An example of the experiential learning cycle in use

In this example, practical nursing experience has been followed by reflection on that experience. Out of that reflective process has evolved a variety of theoretical and conceptual issues which have led the nurse to further study. New learning has then been carried over into practical experience and thus the cycle has been continued. Throughout the process, experience leads to new knowledge and that new knowledge informs practice.

A major factor in the use of the experiential learning cycle is the development of the self-reflective ability used in Stage 2 of the cycle. Much of life is lived without *noticing* what is being thought or felt. For the experiential learning cyle to work individuals must notice themselves and become more aware of what they are doing. Such awareness takes concentration and patience, but once mastered can become a useful tool for living. It can be enhanced through practices such as meditation and co-counselling (Bond 1986; Burnard 1985a), both of which improve the ability to concentrate and to pay attention. Courses in these methods are frequently offered by extra-mural departments of colleges and universities.

Thus, the means by which the nurse may 'take every reasonable opportunity to maintain and improve professional knowledge and competance' may be summarised as follows. There should be an appreciation for the need for lifelong education both by nurse educators and by individual practitioners. Responsibility for learning may be taken by all nurses once they have established a basic knowledge and skills base. There may have to be a gradual move from a 'classical' curriculum towards a 'romantic' curriculum. Again, the individual nurse can gain much from considering the principles of such a curriculum. All nurses need to develop a reflective ability that makes them aware of their own thoughts, feelings and actions. Such reflection can be an important method of modifying future nursing practice. A person cannot *do* anything about himself until he *knows* something about himself. Such knowledge can come through regular use of the experiential learning cycle. Thus, professional knowledge and competence starts with *personal* knowledge and competence and this theme is developed further in the next chapter.

REFERENCES

Bond, M. (1986) *Stress and Self-Awareness: A Guide for Nurses.* Heinemann: London.
Burnard, P. (1985a) Future Imperfect? *Senior Nurse,* 2:1, 8-10.

Burnard, P. (1985b) *Learning Human Skills: A Guide for Nurses.* Heinemann: London.

Burnard, P. (1987) Self and Peer Assessment. *Senior Nurse,* **6:** 5, 16-17.

Freire, P. (1980) *Cultural Action for Freedom.* Penguin: Harmondsworth.

Jarvis, P. (1983a) *The Theory and Practice of Adult and Continuing Education.* Croom Helm: London.

Jarvis, P. (1983b) *The Sociology of Adult and Continuing Education.* Croom Helm: London.

Heron, J. (1973) *Experiential Training Techniques: Human Potential Research Project.* University of Surrey: Guildford.

Kagan, C. et al. (1986) *Interpersonal Skills Training for Nurses:* An Experiential Approach. Harper and Row: London.

Kilty, J. (1981) *Self and Peer Assessment: Human Potential Research Project.* University of Surrey: Guildford.

Knowles, M. (1981) *The Adult Learner: a Neglected Species* (2nd ed). Gulf: Texas.

Lawton, D. (1973) *Social Change, Educational Theory and Curriculum Planning.* Hodder and Stoughton: London.

Peters, R.S. (1969) *Ethics and Education.* Allen and Unwin: London.

Pirsig, R. (1976) *Zen and the Art of Motorcyle Maintenance.* Arrow: London.

Rogers, C. R. (1983) *Freedom to Learn for the Eighties.* Merrill: Columbus, Ohio.

UKCC (1986) *Project 2000.* United Kingdom Central Council for Nursing Midwifery and Health Visiting: London.

Whitehead, A. N. (1932) *The Aims of Education.* Benn: London.

CHAPTER 4

Knowing your Limitations

*Acknowledge any limitations of competence and refuse in
such cases to accept delegated functions without first having
received instruction in regard to those functions and having
been assessed as competent.*

Nurses must know their limits: they must have a firm understanding of what they do know and what they do not: what skills they
have and what skills they lack. In order to appreciate limits it is
necessary to develop self-awareness. But what is self-awareness and
how can it be developed? In order to answer these questions it may
be helpful to identify those aspects that go to make up a concept
of self.

Developing the work of Carl Jung (1983), five aspects of the self can
be identified:

–Sensing.
–Thinking.
–Feeling.
–Intuiting.
–Body experience.

These five aspects of the self will now be considered and methods
identified for developing awareness in each of them. It should be
acknowledged that this is only one way of analysing the concept of
self. The concept is a complicated one that has been debated by
philosophers, theologians, psychologists and sociologists for
centuries. What is important here is that a concrete and usable
concept of self may be useful in nursing. (For other concepts and

discussions of the question of self, the reader is referred to Rogers (1951), Williams (1973), Canfield and Wells (1976), and Macquarrie (1973).)

The first four domains of the self identified above refer to internal psychological aspects. Jung summarises concisely the function of each of these aspects:

> The essential function of sensation is to establish that something exists, thinking tells us what it means, feeling what its value is and intuition surmises whence it comes and wither it goes. (Jung 1983).

The first aspect, then, is sensation. It is arguable that everything that is thought about or felt is experienced first through one or more of the five special senses: hearing, seeing, tasting, touching or smelling, of which the first two are perhaps the most highly developed. In order that the individual can make sense of the world at all, that world must first be experienced via the senses.

It is easy, however, for attention to the senses to be lost. Very often a person is so distracted by his thoughts and feelings that he fails to pay full attention to what they or hears. In this way the person fails to take full advantage of an educational encounter or, alternatively, a considerable amount of a patient's communication is lost. In order to appreciate fully the inputs that are being received through the senses, a person must concentrate on them. A simple experiment may serve to drive this point home. Stop reading this book for a moment and pay close attention to what you can hear around you. As you do so, you will suddenly notice how much auditory input has been filtered out prior to undertaking the experiment. Such filtering-out is essential at times, but at others it is necessary to resist this shutting-off process and pay close attention to what is going on around.

Part of becoming more self-aware is the process of 'noticing': simply paying attention to what is being seen and heard. The development of such attention can help to ensure greater accuracy of reporting, greater observational skill and a greater resistance to making snap judgements and evaluations. People who pay conscious attention to what they see or hear gather accurate data and therefore are in a better position to make considered judgements. Such a position is in line with the Code of Conduct's requirement that the nurses acknowledge their limitations of competence.

Once information enters through one of the senses, it is *thought* about. Thinking here refers to the processes of puzzling, pondering, analysing and criticising. It is essential that people should reflect upon *what* they know, on whether or not what they know is accurate and what they need to *develop* in terms of knowledge. In this sense, it is necessary to develop a continuous and consistent ability to be critical: regularly to question what is held to be true. This is not a comfortable process! It is sometimes far easier to hang on to an old set of beliefs that has been useful in the past than to question the validity of those beliefs. It is far less comfortable, still, to adopt Marx's favourite maxim 'Doubt everything!' (Singer 1980). This inner reflection on knowledge and upon its validity and present-day utility value is, again, part of the requirement being proposed by the Code of Conduct. To acknowledge limitations and to refuse to accept certain delegated functions is to have pondered first upon one's own knowledge and skills base.

The next aspect of the self is feelings. The term feelings here refers to the whole spectrum of emotions, ranging on the one hand from elation to profound depression, on the other. What is important is that the individual learns to develop the ability to identify and acknowledge her feelings in a given situation. In nursing it is often far easier (and sometimes encouraged) either to ignore or rationalise feelings as they occur in day-to-day practice and even to pretend that they simply do not exist. This is evident in the image of the nurse as an implacable, objective carer who has somehow learned to detach herself from emotion. Quite how this image has developed over the years is unclear but its effects are well documented by Bond (1986). She points out that consistent bottling up of emotion can lead to frustration, anxiety and to burn-out – i.e. total disenchantment with the process of nursing and caring.

Heron (1977) notes that, amongst other things, the bottling up of feelings in this way can lead to:

- *Physical tension*, with resultant muscular tension and postural problems.
- *Mental blocks* and the inability to concentrate and make decisions.
- *Emotional numbness*: the inability to express *any* sorts of positive
- feelings – love, caring, affection and so forth.
- *Emotional outbursts*, where the bottled-up emotion suddenly rushes to the surface and manifests itself as outbursts of tears or anger.

Heron offers a comprehensive account of how emotions become

bottled up through the process of living and how emotional release can lead to clearer thinking and more rational decision-making.

To attempt to bottle up feelings in this way is also a strategy that rarely works completely, as emotional feelings are usually 'given away' by facial expression, tone of voice, choice of words, use of metaphors, hand gestures, and so forth (Argyle 1976; Bandler and Grinder 1982). We are always communicating – even when we think that we have succesfully camouflaged our feelings, they tend to reveal themselves! Now what is being advocated here is not that nurses should disclose all their feelings to patients but that it is helpful to all relationships if feelings can be identified by the individual as they occur. If such identification can take place and the person, through reflection, can acknowledge how she feels, then the range of the individual's *choice* increases. Once feelings have been identified, the individual has at least the following choices:

- –To express them.
- –To ignore them.
- –To deal with them later.

If no such identification of feelings occurs, no such range of choices exists.

If, through acting in this reflective way, the individual decides to deal with her feelings later, a number of other options become available. At some time later, those feelings can be talked-through with a friend or a colleague. Alternatively, a more structured approach such as co-counselling can be used (Heron 1974; 1978).

Co-counselling courses are offered by a number of university extra-mural departments and by many further and higher education colleges. Co-counselling has also been advocated as a peer-support strategy in nurse education (Kilty 1983). In essence, the method requires that two people, trained in co-counselling, should meet for an allotted time. They spend half of that time in the role of counsellor to the other's client, and then switch roles for the other half. In this way, both people receive equal amounts of time to talk through problems, express pent-up feelings and design new coping strategies. It is important to note, however, that in co-counselling the role of 'client' is the most important one and the person occupying the role of 'counsellor' does not counsel in the traditional sense of the word. They do not offer advice nor make suggestions on how the other person may 'put her life right'. Instead, they act more as a 'sounding board' for the client who, in this relationship, soon learns to 'counsel herself'. In this sense, then, the client in the co-counselling relationship retains autonomy and does not become dependent on the counsellor.

Other options available to the person who decides to deal with emotions later, include the use of meditation (Le Shan 1974; Hewitt 1978), and the transmutation of strong emotion through sport or exercise. A further range of methods of coping with emotions is offered by Bond (1986) and with particular reference to nurses. Decisions about how a particular individual copes with stress are often matters of personal preference, personality type and practical considerations such as time and resources. It is remarkable, however, how frequently the nurse 'puts off' the process of dealing practically with stress, claiming to be 'too busy'!

Given the stressful nature of nursing and the fact that even very junior nurses are frequently called upon to look after people in particularly difficult circumstances, it would seem reasonable to suggest that the domain of feelings needs addressing more fully in both clinical and educational circles. The profession cannot afford to carry on as though nurses were somehow detached emotionally. Human suffering always calls for involvement, and involvement in the human condition always includes feelings. To ignore the domain of feelings in nurses is to ignore an important part of what it means to be a human being.

The fourth aspect of the self is the intuitive domain. Intuition refers to a hunch or notion that may occur apparently independently of the senses: it is as if we know something to be the case without our necessarily having confirming evidence for it. Now, such intuition may be explained away in terms of some elaborate cognitive process that is yet to be understood or, for some, it may be thought of as some sort of unconscious process. For others, it has mystical connotations. However it is explained and whatever theories are offered for it, it does appear to be an important phenomenon. Indeed, the counsellor and therapist Carl Rogers argued that he was functioning at his most therapeutically when he paid attention to and acted upon his intuitive feelings during a counselling session (Rogers 1967). In the nursing field, Benner (1984) argues from her research that very skilled nursing practitioners often make decisions about nursing intervention intuitively.

The argument here is that the nurse needs to pay attention to this intuitive apect as an important part of self-awareness. It is these sudden intuitive ideas that occur during conversations with patients that can lead to useful problem-solving and important changes in care. This aspect of care might be called the 'artistic' side as compared to the 'scientific' side, which tends to remain firmly rooted in the cognitive and rational domain. Equally important, however, is the need to balance such intuition with a calm, rational and logical approach to work and care. Just as we cannot always deliver thorough and systematic care through appealing only to logic and science, neither can we rely only on intuition. Indeed, Jung (1983) argued that the self-aware person was the one who could *balance* the four aspects of mind: thinking, feeling, sensing and intuiting, for all are important.

A final aspect of self is body experience. It is possible to talk about the body as if it were separate from the rest of the person. Thus it is not uncommon to hear people use expressions such as 'I don't like my body' or 'I'm not happy with my body', as though it were some sort of appendage! To talk of a self-concept must be to include a bodily sense of self. Thus, part of developing self-awareness is developing an accurate body image and perhaps a sense of responsibility for the body. In recent years, nurses have become increasingly aware of the part they play in acting as positive role-models in the campaign against smoking, and it is notable that the Royal College of Nursing has a policy of no smoking on its premises. It would appear, then, that in matters of physical health and appearance, nurses should also pay attention to how they present themselves to the public. Christine Hancock makes this point rather forcibly when she says: 'We are often saying publicly we claim to believe in health but really we like ill health, sickness and early death.' (Hancock 1987). She goes on to argue that nurses must improve their presentation of self to the public. Part of this process begins with the individual's awareness of her own body, its appearance and its capabilities. Again, this is in keeping with the fourth statement of the Code of Conduct. Part of competence and appreciating limits is an awareness of one's own physical strength (or lack of it), agility and ability to exercise psychomotor dexterity. Further, the more psychological aspects of self are perhaps mediated by our physical sense of self. Thus our internal self-image is usually improved by a confident and healthy external presentation. There are, of course, numerous methods of increasing the physical sense of well-being, ranging from exercise and diet to specific sporting and recreational activities.

This, then, is an approach to understanding the concepts of self and self-awareness. Such awareness is a necessary prerequisite of any decision-making about whether or not to accept delegated instructions in nursing practice. Once we are aware of our abilities and shortcomings, we are in a position to do something about them.

Without such awareness, we are 'blind' and because of this blindness probably less effective in our delivery of care.

Once limitations have been discovered, the next stage is to rectify them. This is where the notion of self-directed learning alluded to in the previous chapter is particularly appropriate. Malcolm Knowles (1975) advocates the use of personal learning contracts. Such a contract can be designed by an individual nurse in co-operation with a nurse tutor or a lecturer. Alternatively, the contract can be written out for its own sake as a method of clarifying learning objectives and methods of evaluation. Thirdly, it can be used in the clinical setting as part of a learning programme or as an aspect of staff development. Figure 4.1 identifies the outline of a learning contract and offers an example of its use. Such a contract identifies learning objectives, learning resources and evaluation methods in such a way as to ensure that a thorough educational experience is undertaken.

LEARNING CONTRACT

Name: John Doe   Learning Project: Applying the Nursing
                                  Process in Psychiatric Nursing

1 Learning Objectives	2 Learning Resources and Strategies	3 Evidence of Accomplishment	4 Criteria and Means of Validating Evidence
1 To define the nursing process	– the library – the School of Nursing – nursing journals	A short essay on the nursing process	Presentation of the essay at a ward meeting attended by a clinical teacher
2 To use the nursing process in planning the care of two patients	– the charge nurse – the clinical teacher - books on the subject	Two care plans written out in the patients' notes	Rating of the care plans by two peers and by the clinical teacher and charge nurse

Figure 4.1 An example of a learning contract

By regular use of a learning contract and through maintenance and development of self-awareness, the nurse can monitor her own performance in terms of Statement Four of the Code of Conduct.

Limitations of competence can be the basis from which to move forward and to develop an ever-widening range of skills and knowledge. Such development is in keeping with present-day educational theory which stresses the need for continuing and lifelong education (Jarvis 1983). No longer can basic nurse training be expected to serve the nurse throughout her career nor can nurse education remain an impartial knowledge-based process. Today, it is vital that self-knowledge be incorporated into this lifelong process of learning to nurse.

REFERENCES

Argyle, M. (1976) *The Psychology of Interpersonal Behaviour.* Penguin: Harmondsworth.

Bandler, R. and Grinder, J. (1982) *Reframing: Neurolinguistic Programming and the Transformation of Meaning.* Real People Press: Moab, Utah.

Benner, P. (1984) *From Novice to Expert: Excellence and Power in Clinical Nursing Practice.* Addison-Wesley: Menlo Park, California.

Bond, M. (1986) *Stress and Self-Awareness: a Guide for Nurses.* Heinemann: London.

Canfield, J. and Wells, H.C. (1976) *100 Ways to Enhance Self-concept in the Classroom.* Prentice-Hall: Englewood Cliffs, New Jersey.

Hancock, C. (1987) Generally Speaking. *Senior Nurse:* **6:**4: 8-9.

Heron, J. (1974) *Reciprocal Counselling Manual.* Human Potential Research Project, University of Surrey: Guildford.

Heron, J. (1977) *Catharsis in Human Development.* Human Potential Research Project, University of Surrey: Guildford.

Heron, J. (1978) *Co-Counsellor's Teacher's Manual.* Human Potential Research Project, University of Surrey: Guildford.

Hewitt, J. (1978) *Meditation.* Hodder and Stoughton: Sevenoaks, Kent.

Jung, C.G. (1983) *Selected Writings.* (ed. A. Storr). Pan: London.

Kilty, J. (1983) *Experiential Learning: Human Potential Research Project.* University of Surrey: Guildford.

Knowles, M. (1975) *Self-directed Learning: A guide for learners and teachers.* Cambridge: New York.

Le Shan, M. (1974) *How to Meditate.* Turnstone Press: Wellingborough.

Macquarrie, J. (1973) *Existentialism.* Penguin: Harmondsworth.

Rogers, C.R. (1951) *Client-centred Counselling.* Constable, London.

Rogers, C.R. (1967) *On Becoming a Person.* Constable: London.

Singer, P. (1980) *Marx.* Oxford University Press: Oxford.

Williams, B. (1973) *The Problem of Self.* Cambridge University Press: Cambridge.

CHAPTER 5

Working Together

Work in a collaborative and co-operative manner with other health care professionals and recognise and respect their particular contributions within the health care team.

The explosion of knowledge that has occurred during this century has made it impossible for one person to possess all the knowledge and skill required to treat the sick in society. This has resulted in the emergence of new professional groups, many of them, such as physiotherapy and radiography, having evolved from tasks at one time included in nursing. While this has enabled highly qualified and skilled practitioners to deal with specific aspects of patient care it has also meant that teams of people have had to come together to ensure that all aspects of care are adequately covered.

Working in a team is therefore a common experience for today's health professionals and one with which all nurses are familiar. A typical ward team will comprise a ward sister or charge nurse, other qualified nurses (staff nurses), learners, physiotherapists, possibly physiotherapy students, a social worker, perhaps a speech therapist and others. There will also be the medical staff: consultant physicians or surgeons, registrars, house officers and medical students attached to the 'firm'. In addition, there may be a ward clerk, a ward receptionist, auxillaries and domestic workers – a formidable array of people, all there ostensibly to 'care for the patient'.

However, this apparently common goal may not be perceived as important in the short term by any of the people involved. The medical consultant may be concerned to demonstrate efficiency by achieving a high bed occupancy. The ward domestic may have as her goal the most highly polished floors in the hospital; the student nurse may want the opportunity to carry out new techniques; the medical student wants interesting cases, and so on. None of these goals is necessarily bad in itself provided the needs of the patients remain paramount, and this can be achieved by good leadership. But who is the leader of this team? The medical consultant may consider that as it is normally a medical decision to admit or discharge patients that the team leader must be a doctor, yet the ward sister is frequently described as the co-ordinator of care and that may be considered as a leadership role. For a patient whose main aim is to learn to walk again after illness the physiotherapist may seem to be the key person. Research into the continuity of care of geriatric patients identified the fact that personalised care under the authority of the nurse resulted in a more effective regime than care under the control of the doctor. Experimental National Health Nursing Homes and units within the Oxford Regional Health Authority have utilised this approach. In these places the nurse has the authority to both admit and discharge the patient and to call in medical staff when needed on a true 'consultancy' basis. In this case the nurse is obviously the team leader.

What is essential is that each individual should recognise the contribution that can be made by the others involved in the care of patients so that the most appropriate skills are utilised. Competition is not the most effective way to ensure that the goals relating to patient cure and care are best achieved, as the Code states the nurse should 'Work in a collaborative and co-operative manner with other health care professionals and recognise and respect their particular contribution within the health care team'. Although this phrase specifies fellow 'professionals' no discussion on team work in health care can ignore the contribution of relatives, voluntary workers and indeed the patient or client as part of the team.

There is a real danger that once a person becomes a patient the health care team feel that they 'possess' that individual and that as a patient he has to surrender all 'rights' to them. This is not so: the patient, or if he is unable to express an opinion by reason of illness or handicap, a relative or guardian, has the right to information about his treatment and care, to understand the prognosis, to appreciate the possible side-effects of treatment and to be made aware of alternative strategies. When this information has been made available, it still remains the patient's prerogative to accept or decline the treatment and care offered or to decline it is still the prerogative of the patient.

The American Hospital Association has formulated A Patient's Bill of Rights (1973):

1. The patient has the right to considerate and respectful care.
2. The patient has the right to obtain from his physician complete current information concerning his diagnosis, treatment and prognosis in terms the patient can reasonably be expected to understand. When it is not medically advisable to give such information to the patient, the information should be made available to an appropriate person on his behalf. He has the right to know, by name, the physician responsible for co-ordinating his care.
3. The patient has the right to receive from his physician information necessary to give informed consent prior to the start of any procedure and/or treatment. Except in emergencies, such information for informed consent should include but not necessarily be limited to the specific procedure and/or treatment, the medically significant risks involved, and the probable duration of incapacitation. Where medically significant alternatives for care or treatment exist, or where the patient requests information concerning medical alternatives, the patient has the right to such information. The patient also has the right to know the name of the person responsible for the procedures or treatment.
4. The patient has the right to refuse treatment to the extent permitted by law, and to be informed of the medical consequences of his action.
5. The patient has the right to every consideration of his privacy concerning his own medical care programme. Case discussion, consultation, examination and treatment are confidential and should be conducted discreetly. Those not directly involved in his care must have the permission of the patient to be present.
6. The patient has the right to expect that all communications and records pertaining to his care should be treated as confidential.
7. The patient has the right to expect that within its capacity a hospital must make reasonable response to the request of a patient for services. The hospital must provide evaluation, service and/or referral as indicated by the urgency of the case. When medically permissible a patient may be transferred to another facility only after he has received complete information and full explanation concerning the need for and alternatives to such a transfer. The institution to which the patient is to be transferred must first have accepted the patient for transfer.
8. The patient has the right to obtain information as to any relationship of his hospital to other health care and educational in-

stitutions in so far as his care is concerned. The patient has the right to obtain information as to the existence of any professional relationship among individuals, by name, who are treating him.

9. The patient has the right to be advised if the hospital proposes to engage in or perform human experimentation affecting his care or treatment. The patient has the right to refuse to participate in such research projects.

10. The patient has the right to expect reasonable continuity of care. He has the right to know in advance what appointment times and physicians are available, and where. The patient has the right to expect that the hospital will provide a mechanism whereby he is informed by his physician or a delegate of the physician of the patient's continuing health care requirements following discharge.

11. The patient has the right to examine and receive an explanation of his bill regardless of the source of payment.

12. The patient has the right to know what hospital rules and regulations apply to his conduct as a patient.

This Bill makes it quite explicit that the patient has to be considered as an equal part of the health care team concerned with his welfare, and although it refers to hospital patients the principles can and should be applied to patients and clients receiving care in the community.

Many health care professionals pay lip service to these rights but still feel that, because of their position, superior knowledge and/or skill, that their views should carry more weight.

The problem of paternalism, or perhaps more accurately parentalism, is an ever-present one in the health care setting. There is an implicit expectation amongst most health care professionals that the patient or client by entering the health care institution has surrendered all powers of intellect and has become in effect 'a little child'. Tied in with this is the somewhat Victorian attitude that 'children should be seen and not heard' – hence, the all too frequent complaint made by patients that the doctors or nurses not only did not explain the situation to them or consult them, but in many cases they talked over them as if they did not exist. Linked with this approach is the view that the professional must know what is best for the patient or client and therefore should be obeyed. Such an approach is deeply resented by many patients who ask, quite rightly, 'Whose life is it ?' Unfortunately, many patients lack the confidence or the assertiveness to question doctors' decisions or to disagree with them. Quiet compliance is often the unhappy position adopted by many people when they become patients.

The question may be raised here of whether all team members are of equal worth. The answer to this question raises another – equal in what sense? Obviously, not all have the same knowledge or skill: some will have different attitudes and, as has already been discussed, individual goals may vary. Nevertheless, if all are needed for the effective care of the patient then all should be equally valued for their contribution. The Apostle Paul expressed this most succinctly when considering the part played by the members of the Church in Corinth. He compared the Church to the human body in which each part is different yet all are essential to the full and effective functioning of the person: 'If all were one part, where would the body be?' As it is there are many parts but one body. The eye cannot say to the hand 'I don't need you!' And the head cannot say to the feet 'I don't need you!' On the contrary, those parts of the body that seem to be weaker are indispensable – so there should be no division in the body, but its parts should have equal concern for each other.

The doctor has often been accorded supremacy within the team, in part due to the fact that, as already discussed, it is often a medical prerogative to admit and discharge patients; however, there are other factors which tend to ensure that the doctor is seen to be more important than the other team members. One important factor is that, until recently, the doctor has been the only member of the team who has had the benefit of higher education and, hence, other team members including nurses have felt unable to challenge the doctor's views on the way in which patients are perceived and/or treated. That situation is changing and one of the comments made about nurses who have taken a degree in nursing is that they are not afraid to question decisions made by the medical members of the team. The fact that, traditionally, doctors were men and nurses women has also had an effect on the way they perceived each other and that, coupled with the generally higher social class of the doctor compared with the nurse, has further served to enhance doctors' status. Once again the situation is changing. There are now many women in medicine and an increasing number of men in nursing. These factors may help to change traditional attitudes and ensure that people are accorded the respect and status that they earn rather than have their position in the team ascribed to them by virtue of the role that they fill.

Occasionally, conflict occurs within teams, usually due to the team members holding different goals or values regarding care and cure.

Sometimes these values are related to fundamental issues such as the practice of euthanasia, abortion or genetic engineering. In these cases open and honest discussion between all members of the team, including the patient, is essential; and where agreement cannot be reached, and the law does not provide guidance, provision must be made for conscientious objection so that any individual team member can withdraw from the situation. In one sense, it is important that the individual is seen to be accountable to his or her self – this requires the person to be able to make decisions regarding actions that enable the person to 'live with him or herself'. The right to make a stand on conscientious grounds should be possible without any organisational or professional repercussion. To ensure the safety of the patient, the individual should ensure that his or her views are known in advance so that withdrawal is anticipated.

One of the benefits of teamwork is that a new member of the team may receive support from more experienced members who will provide the novice with a variety of role-models. Not that learning is restricted to the new member – all team members can and should learn from each other. This is as true for the patient as for the professionals: what is required from all is honesty, trust in each other and a respect for the contribution made by each individual.

REFERENCES

American Hospital Association (1973) *A Patient's Bill of Rights*.
Paul 1 Corinthians 12: 19-23.

CHAPTER 6

Customs, Values and Spiritual Beliefs

Take account of the customs, values and spiritual beliefs of patients/clients.

We live in a multiracial, multicultural society. Statement Six of the code requires that nurses take account of the customs, values and spiritual beliefs of patients or clients.

Customs are a person's regular or established ways of behaving. They are often linked to that person's country of birth, upbringing, life experience and belief systems. For some, customs are so ingrained that they are carried out unconsciously, others (and particularly if they are linked to a particular spiritual belief or value system) are very precisely carried out with attention to ritual. Because customs of any sort are embedded so deeply in the background and experience of the person it is important that the nurse respects individual differences, for to question a person's customs is to question that person's self-concept.

A problem arises here as to how nurses can *recognise* other people's customs. Sometimes the behaviour of other people, if it is unusual, may seem unintelligable or irrational. If this is the case, then it is easy to dismiss that person's customs as odd behaviour. What is perhaps essential, is that nurses should develop (a) a background knowledge of a variety of examples of customs that relate to particular groups of people, and (b) an understanding of and perspective on their own customs.

In order to develop an understanding of the variety of customs that relate to particular groups of people it is necessary to draw on a number of sources. A short list would include: anthropology, geography, sociology, psychology and theology. Anthropology can help in placing people in a particular cultural and social situation (Fox 1975) and can aid in developing a deep perspective on different styles and ways of living together in a particular country or culture. Geography gives clues as to particular lifestyles based on location in the physical world – for example, life in a mountainous areas or in low temperatures. Sociology offers an analysis, and possibly an explanation, of how and why people form groups, co-operate, fight and generally exist in a state of interdependence (Chapman 1977). Psychology offers a closer focus on the individual and suggests a variety of theories about the nature of individual thinking, feeling and behaving. It must be borne in mind, however, that much of the sociological and psychological literature is *western* in its orientation: the degree to which such western thinking can readily accommodate cultural differences is an open question. In other words, can a theorist working and thinking in the West truly understand and account for the behaviour and customs of those living in the East?

Finally, theology can explain some of the significance of custom from a religious point of view. Again, the temptation to view 'our' view of religion as the 'right' one needs to be resisted here. This, of course, poses something of a problem. If a particular set of beliefs is held to be 'true', it is naturally difficult to accept that another set of beliefs may also be 'true'! The ability to acknowledge and accept such ambiguity may be a clear sign of open-mindedness and wisdom.

All these disciplines offer different kinds of analysis of human action from different perspectives. The skilled nurse would do well to consider these various perspectives as an aid to developing a rich background from which to view *this* patient's behaviour and customs at *this* time. For human action never occurs in isolation, it is always embedded in the particular social and psychological context prevalent at the time.

If time is taken to absorb some of the ideas that can be gained from the disciplines outlined above, those ideas can be used to enable the nurse to clarify her own customs. The questions here are 'Why do I act in the way that I do, and how did I come to adopt these patterns of behaviour?' To answer these questions requires some knowledge of the sociological concept of socialisation and of the psychological process known as introjection. Reflection and introspection are also required.

The first stage in the reflective process is becoming conscious of the fact that we act at all. This may seem a ludicrous statement: surely we all *know* that we act? A moment's reflection, however, will probably reveal that we do not often *notice* how we act. Much of our action happens spontaneously and without forethought or attention. What is being suggested here is a willing and conscious attention to what is done and why. Heron (1977) has referred to this process as 'conscious use of the self'. Once a person begins to notice consciously what is done, it is easier to identify reasons for doing it.

Having begun this process of noticing, it is then possible to compare that action with the theories or explanations offered for human behaviour by anthropologists, sociologists, psychologists and theologians. In this way we can 'personalise' the theories and come to develop theories about personal behaviour, based on rational thought. This reflective and comparative process can lead to an enhanced degree of self-understanding, without which it is impossible to understand the behaviour and customs of others.

The process of valuing or holding values, consists, according to Raths, Harmin and Sidney (1966), of three sub-processes: (a) prizing one's own beliefs and behaviours, (b) choosing those beliefs and behaviours, and (c) acting on those beliefs. Like customs, values are deeply grounded in cultural heritage, experience and personal belief systems. Also, like customs, they are part of a person's self-concept: those beliefs or behaviours that are held as important (or valuable) *make* the individual. Values are things that modify behaviour through a process of self-monitoring. Personal value systems allow or disallow certain actions. As with customs, values vary from culture to culture, from group to group and from person to person, and it can never be assumed that other people's value systems are similar to ours. Thus, in nursing, respect for other people's values is vital.

The process of self-reflection and introspection can again help us to identify our values. An aid to this process is a series of exercises in values-clarification offered by Simon, Howe and Kirschenbaum (1978). They argue that many people are unaware of their own value systems and therefore have difficulty in knowing how to make decisions about how to act. Through clearly identifying our values we are better equipped to make decisions about how to live our lives. We are also in a better position to appreciate the difference between *our* value system and other people's.

It is, of course, one thing to identify and clarify personal values and quite another to appreciate the effect of that value system on other people. Values are reflected in most of the things that are done and, particularly, in the way things are said: hence the need to develop the facility of paying attention to our verbal behaviour in order that our value system does not offend other people. Consider, for instance, the following situations:

- The patient who tells you that he has 'no religion' when an initial nursing process assessment is being made.
- The patient admitted with AIDS who talks to you about his gay partner.
- The unmarried adolescent girl who is admitted because of complications during pregnancy.

In each of these situations, what is said to the patient will reflect a particular value system. Notice that it is impossible to escape from the valuing process. For instance, it may be acknowledged in the above cases that the life situation of each person is acceptable. On the other hand, some or all of these lifestyles may be unacceptable. Whether 'accepted' or not, a particular value statement is made. In this sense, there is no neutral ground. What is important, however, is the acknowledgement that *whatever* position one holds, that of other people is equally valid. A nurse is on difficult ground if she condemns others for the values that they hold and on even more difficult ground if that condemnation is verbalised. Such behaviour is not in keeping with the Code of Conduct nor with the process of caring for others.

Linked to the question of values is that of spiritual beliefs. In order for nurses to consider thoughtfully other people's spiritual beliefs it is important that they appreciate the basic differences between different sorts of faiths, and, indeed, ways of living *without* a set of religious beliefs – atheism, agnosticism and secular humanism. Spiritual issues have been defined elswhere as those that are concerned with personal meaning or how we make sense of the world around us (Burnard 1987). That meaning may be framed in religious terms or it may not. The person who adopts an atheistic, agnostic or secular humanistic position is still creating meaning: it is just that such meaning does not necessarily include a concept of God. It is worth considering, then, the basic tenets of the major religions of the world and the non-religious philosophies that enable people to create meaning.

Whilst Christianity can be divided into (at least) the Orthodox Church, the Protestant Churches and the Roman Catholic Church, there are certain tenets of faith that are common to all three. Within each of the main divisions also exist a wide range of different sects and denominations. All major Christian churches believe in the historical significance of Jesus of Nazareth as the son of God, born of a virgin. The essence of Christianity can be identified in the Apostles' Creed:

> I believe in God the Father Almighty, Creator of heaven and earth: and in Jesus Christ his only Son, our Lord who was conceived by the Holy Spirit, born of the Virgin Mary: suffered under Pontius Pilate, was crucified, dead and buried, he descended into hell; the third day he rose again from the dead and ascended into heaven; is seated at the right hand of God the Father Almighty; from thence he shall come to judge the quick and the dead. I believe in the Holy Ghost; the holy Catholic Church; the Communion of Saints; the forgiveness of sins; the Resurrection of the body, and the life of the world to come. Amen.

The word 'Catholic' in this passage refers to the notion of universality and is not synonymous with the Roman Catholic Church. Christians of all denominations (and a great many of them are described by Sampson:1982), celebrate the following principal festivals: Christmas, Lent, Good Friday, Easter Sunday and Whitsun (Pentecost). However, there are a great number of variations of practice in individual denominations and sects. It cannot be assumed that all Christians believe the same things beyond the basic tenets identified above. The theological and doctrinal position adopted by different denominations varies greatly, as does the attention paid to the role of ritual and ceremony. These variations are vitally important to individual believers and are well articulated by Sampson (1982) and Rumbold (1986).

Judaism is a religion essentially of a particular people, the Jews. The history of Judaism and much more of its theological basis can be found in the Old Testament of the Holy Bible. The Law of the Jewish people is written in the Torah, or first five books of the Old Testament. They await the Messiah and do not recognise Jesus of Nazareth as that Messiah. Important Jewish festivals include: Rosh Hashanah (Jewish New Year), Yom Kippur (the Day of Atonement), Succoth (Feast of Tabernacles), Simchath Torah (Rejoicing in the Law), Chanukah (the Feast of Esther), Purim (the Feast of Lots), Pesach (the Passover) and Tishah B'Av (Mourning for the Destruction of the Temple). Orthodox Jews require their food to be prepared following a specific ritual, and abstain from certain types of meat, notably pork.

Hinduism is an ancient religion originally centred in India and Nepal but which has spread wherever Indians have settled. Hindus

believe that there are many gods but that all of these are manifest-
ations of one God. Hinduism has no fixed creed and is a very diverse
religion. There are a variety of schools of Hindu philosophy and a
number of separate religions have developed from it, including
Buddhism. In the Hindu religion the cow is regarded as a sacred
animal and therefore beef is not eaten.

The religion of Islam is followed by Muslims. Islam literally means
submission and Muslims are committed to submitting themselves
to the will of Allah. In the Islamic faith, Muslims believe Him to be
the one true God. They consider Mohammed to be the last great
prophet following chronologically after the Jewish prophets and
Jesus Christ, and they follow his teachings. Again, for Muslims
animals used for food have to be slaughtered in a ritual manner.

Clearly, this cannot claim to be an exhaustive description of the
religions under discussion nor does it claim to be a comprehensive
listing of all the world's religions. As we have noted, there is already
a considerable literature on the topic to which the reader is referred.
It is important in this context, however, to note the considerable
differences between the ways in which different cultures give meaning to religious experience. Given the multicultural nature of our
society, it is important that all nurses have some appreciation of
these different religious interpretations and respect the differences
between them.

Finally, we may consider the issues of atheism and agnosticism.
Both are dimensions of spirituality in that both are aspects of some
people's belief systems or their attempts to create meaning. Both
may be equally respected in the manner that 'religious' beliefs are
respected.

Atheism is the unequivocal denial of the possible existence of God.
The atheist is the 'unbeliever', the person who does not believe in
God. It is interesting to ponder on our individual reaction to such a
position. For instance, it is possible to respond by seeing such a
person as 'wrong', or that such a person needs only to reflect further
for clarification; or that they need more education in order to bring
them to the truth. Or can they be accepted as they are? Various
responses are possible; the least acceptable seems to be the notion
that somehow the believer is 'right' and the unbeliever is 'wrong'.
Belief in God must necessarily involve a 'leap of faith' (Kierkegaard
1959). There can be no ultimate scientific proof of the existence or
non-existence of God. Individuals either believe or do not believe.
Neither does the position of unbelief necessarily preclude any sort

of moral position. An unbeliever is quite as able to lead a moral life as is a believer. Indeed, Simone de Beauvoir argued that unbelievers had to lead a 'more moral' life than believers, for as there is no final arbiter of right and wrong for the unbelievers they are necessarily thrown back on their own decision-making as a guide to conduct. The believer can be 'forgiven': the unbeliever must forgive herself.

Atheists have to look beyond a concept of God for meaning. That they have to do this does not mean that they have no spiritual needs. The spiritual needs of the atheist (in terms of a search for meaning) are just as vital as they are for the believer. Some atheists find that sense of meaning in secular humanism.

Secular humanism should not be confused with 'humanistic psychology' (Shaffer 1978). The base argument of secular humanism is well outlined by Blackham (1968). Briefly, the argument is this: people are alone in that there is no God. Because they are alone, they are responsible for themselves: they also have a joint responsibility for all other persons. In acting for themselves, they should act as though they were acting for all mankind: to do less than this is selfishness and not, so Blackham argues, secular humanism. Such a philosophy offers an immediate sense of meaning: the atheist is responsible for herself and for others. As a result, the 'golden rule' applies: 'treat others as we would wish to be treated'. This, then, is the basis for morality and for meaning without recourse to belief in God.

The agnostic is in a slightly different position. The agnostic argues that because it is impossible to prove or disprove the existence of God, silence on the issue is the only wise position (Bullock and Stallybrass 1977). The agnostic is neither believer or unbeliever, he holds the view that discussion about the matter is necessarily misplaced in the end, because such an issue can only ever be a matter of faith. Again, such a position does not, of itself, rule out the need for meaning or morality. Agnostics, like atheists, still need to discover or invest life with meaning in what they do or how they live. Some may argue that the only meaning that *can* be found in life is that which individuals invest in it (Kopp 1972). In other words, there is no ultimate meaning for the way things are: people bring meaning to their actions. Meaning, therefore, is an intrinsic concept and dependent upon the individual's reasoning or perception.

These are thumbnail sketches of two alternatives to a belief in God. There is, of course, another position, that of the person who either does not know whether or not he believes in God and a further position, that of the person who does not believe such issues to be important. It is argued here that such positions are just as valid as are those adopted by people who would claim to be believers.

There are many situations in which such positions need to be considered in nursing. As we have seen, one of the questions asked on admission of a patient may related to that person's 'religion'. Such a question leaves no doubt that the accepted position is that of 'believer'. Indeed, it is quite possible that many patients in this culture, faced with the question and uncertain about their own beliefs, will answer 'Church of England' or 'Catholic', whether or not they are members of those churches, in order not to embarrass themselves. It may take considerable bravery to answer 'none' or 'atheist' in these circumstances! We need to think long and hard about how we may pose questions of belief or unbelief without making such questions *leading* questions.

Secondly, it is necessary to consider the sorts of value judgement that nurses may make about other people's belief systems. If the nurse is a believer, is there a harsh judgement of the unbeliever? If, on the other hand, the nurse is an unbeliever, is the believer dismissed? It is important that there is an acknowledgement that either belief system may not coincide with that of the patient. Nor is it appropriate that nurses proselytise or evangelise for *either* position. Nurses, in the role of carers, are not required to convert others to belief or unbelief. There are other more delicate questions. Acceptance, for instance of the fact that the unbeliever may not see the need for the conventional funeral service. 'Secular' forms of service are available through national secular societies. It may also need to be acknowledged that death may not be a fearful event for the unbeliever, nor need it be a fearful event for unbelieving relatives.

The whole question of belief and value systems underlies the way nurses approach the issue of patients' spiritual needs. Nurses need, first, to clarify *their own* belief and value systems before they are clearly able to help patients with such 'ultimate' questions. Values clarification exercises may be useful here (Simon, Howe and Kirshenbaum 1978) – so may open discussion in schools of nursing of *all* aspects of spirituality, both religious and secular.

It would do great disservice to a wide variety of ways of addressing spiritual matters if the term 'spiritual' was only connoted as being to do with religious matters. Nurses clearly need to be open minded in their approach to this vital aspect of nursing care.

REFERENCES

Blackham, H.J. (1986) *Humanism.* Pelican: Harmondsworth.

Bullock, A and Stallybrass, O. (eds) (1977) *The Fontana Dictionary of Modern Thought.* Fontana: London.

Burnard, P. (1986) Picking up the pieces. *Nursing Times,* **82:** 17, 37-39.

Burnard, P. (1987) Spiritual Distress and the Nursing Response: Theoretical Considerations and Counselling Skills. *Journal of Advanced Nursing,* **12,** 377-382.

Chapman, C.R. (1977) *Sociology for Nurses:* Baillière Tindall: London.

Fox, R. (1975) *Encounter with Anthropology.* Penguin: Harmondsworth.

Frankl, V. (1963) *Man's Search for Meaning.* Washington Square Books: New York.

Heron, J. (1977) *Behavioural Analysis in Education and Training.* Human Potential Research Project, University of Surrey: Guildford.

Kierkegaard, S. (1959) *Either/Or,* Vol. 1. Doubleday: New York.

Kopp, S. (1972) *If You Meet the Buddha on the Road, Kill Him!: A Modern Pilgrimage Through Myth, Legend, Zen & Psychotherapy.* Sheldon Press: London.

Raths, L. , Harmin, M. and Simon, S. (1966) *Values and Teaching.* Merrill, Columbus, Ohio.

Rumbold, G. (1986) *Ethics in Nursing Practice.* Baillière Tindall: London.

Sampson, C. (1982) *The Neglected Ethic : Religious and Cultural Factors in the Care of Patients.* McGraw-Hill: Maidenhead.

Shaffer, J.P.B. (1978) *Humanistic Psychology.* Prentice-Hall: Englewood Cliffs, New Jersey.

Simon, S., Howe, L.W. and Kirschenbaum, H. (1978) *Values Clarification,* Revised edition. A. and W. Visual Library: New York.

CHAPTER 7

Conscientious Objection

Make known to an appropriate person or authority any conscientious objection which may be relevant to professional practice.

One of the fundamental rights of any person in the United Kingdom is the right to exclusion from any activity on 'conscientious' grounds, Even in wartime, an individual who objects in principle to killing another person may request exemption from military service.

There is an important distinction to be made between an individual who objects to an action because of strongly-held and soundly-based principles and an objection made in a particular situation because at that time there is a conflict of professional judgement. For example, it may be possible for a nurse to consider that in many situations electroconvulsive therapy is a justified treatment but on one specific occasion to consider that the patient is not physically fit to receive this treatment. In this instance, any objection to the patient receiving the treatment is made on professional grounds and may or may not be accepted by the medical staff in charge of the case. Quite a different situation would arise if the nurse objected to the treatment on the ground that it was morally wrong to administer a treatment that interfered with the normal function of the brain. In this case it would be appropriate for that nurse to ask to be relieved from participation in the treatment on conscientious grounds. Obviously, objections based on principle should be made known by the nurse before any specific situation arises so that appropriate staffing arrangements can be made and the patient to be adequately cared for.

The basis for such principles may be religious and/or moral. Such principles have to be decided upon by the individual and cannot be the subject of rules. The philosopher Kant (1785) endeavoured to lay down guidance for individuals who faced the difficult situation of having to decide on the rightness or otherwise of a course of action. He called his guidelines 'categorical imperatives' thus giving them more strength than perhaps many would accord them. The first of these imperatives states that a person should: 'Act only on that maxim through which you can at the same time will that it should become an universal law.'

It is this type of action that is based on a fundamental principle that forms the grounds for conscientious objection. However, it is also expected that a nurse will act in such a way that no harm will befall the patient and therefore it is both morally expected and to a degree required by law that a nurse should make clear any reasons that may exist which indicate to him or her that a proposed course of treatment will not only be of little benefit but may also be harmful to the patient.

It is this type of action that may result in disagreement between health care professionals and which in an ideal world would be resolved by open and frank discussion. However, this is not an ideal world and if the treatment ordered is the responsibility of another professional then the nurse may fail to halt its progress. In such a case it would be wise for the nurse to record the objection made and the grounds for dissent. Such a decision is one for the individual to take and is not one that can be solved by resorting to hierarchical power or policy statements: nevertheless, the nurse lodging an objection may be required to justify the action taken.

The National Board for Nursing, Midwifery and Health Visiting for Scotland issued a Guidance Paper for nurses who objected to a medical treatment, in which it the suggested that the following steps might be helpful:

1. Ask the person who issued the instructions for clarification.
2. The nurse expressing concern should provide factual, rationally defensible evidence for her concern.
3. Clearly documented nursing assessments and records are essential.

All the suggestions in this chapter regarding the nurse being able to *account* for why she wishes to object on conscientious grounds indicate the need for that nurse to identify and understand her own value and belief system. Clearly, people cannot account for why they object to something if they have not given sufficient thought to the basis for their objection. The notion that nurses should become self-aware has been discussed more fully in other parts of this book but it is in the domain of conscientious objection that self-awareness becomes a particularly important prerequisite. It is vital that all nurses should appreciate *what* their beliefs and values are, *why* they hold them, the *limitations* to them, and *areas of likely conflict* either with others or with the profession. Without such clarification, many decisions of conscience may be made 'blindly' and without due rational thought. It is important, in a professional context, that objections should not be made on a whim but be firmly grounded in systematic argument.

Further, it is important that all nurses who wish to object in this way should be able to express their objections clearly and to communicate them appropriately: such expression may be enhanced by nurses developing assertiveness skills (Alberti and Emmons 1982). Assertiveness enables people to be clear about what they want to say, develop the confidence to say it clearly and, if necessary, be prepared to repeat what they have to say. It is arguable that the nursing profession as it exists at present has tended to produce compliant and rather unassertive professionals, and the hierarchical structure of the medical profession and the tradition that the nurse is somewhat lower in status than her medical colleagues has tended to reinforce this self-image. As we have seen, the profession is changing and so is its relationship with medicine: perhaps it is time for nurses to develop assertiveness skills, skills that can easily be taught through the medium of experiential learning. In experiential learning sessions nurses can clarify what it is they have difficulty in saying to others, they can practise being assertive (through role-play and skills rehearsal) and they can receive feedback from their peers as to their effectiveness. Such sessions, if handled well by the facilitator, can increase individual confidence and also make the process of becoming assertive more effective. Like all skills, assertiveness needs practice. Whilst many schools of nursing are currently incorporating the teaching of assertiveness skills into the curriculum, further training is widely available through extramural departments of colleges and universities.

Small groups of nurses may also consider setting up peer support groups in order to learn such skills themselves. Ernst and Goodison (1981) offer a wide range of practical suggestions as to how such a group may be set up, how to keep it going and how to understand and cope with the teething troubles that may arise. Indeed, such a group may serve a triple purpose:

1. To develop assertive skills.
2. To clarify beliefs and values in the company of supportive colleagues.
3. To enhance self-awareness.

All these things will make easier the process of deciding whether or not to object to any aspect of nursing or medicine on conscientious grounds.

REFERENCES

Alberti, R.E. and Emmons, M.L. (1982) *Your Perfect Right: A Guide to Assertive Living*. Impact Publishers: San Luis, California.

Ernst, S. and Goodison, L. (1981) *In Our Own Hands: a book of self-help therapy*. The Women's Press: London.

Kant, I. (1785) *Fundamental Principles of the Metaphysics of Morals*. (Trans. Abbott, T.K.). Library of Literal Arts: New York.

National Board for Nursing, Midwifery and Health Visiting for Scotland. 1985 Guidance Paper. *Questioning of, or objecting to, participation in medical procedures*.

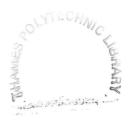

CHAPTER 8

Privileged Relationships

Avoid any abuse of the privileged relationship which exists with patients/clients and of the privileged access allowed to their property, residence or workplace.

The relationship that develops between a patient/client and a health care worker is unique. Unlike the relationships in which individuals normally become involved this is usually one in which neither the patient/client nor the nurse has any real choice. Apart from the situation where an individual engages a specific private nurse the patient has no say as to who is selected to provide care. Equally, the nurse is rarely able to choose the patients allocated to her care or to opt out of involvement. So the situation is one where two individuals who may have little in common socially, or in any other way, find themselves in an intimate interaction.

In addition, the nurse is likely to have access to information not normally disclosed to other people and may be involved in activities that breach customary social taboos. For example, in western society it is not normal for an adult male to be seen naked by a young female except in a close family relationship. The uniqueness of the situation is often remarked upon by older male patients who say, wryly, that the nurse is 'young enough to be my daughter'. Alternatively, many female patients feel embarrassed if examined or cared for by a male doctor or nurse. However, the discomfort is not always experienced by the patient alone as nurses may also feel uneasy in some situations, finding it difficult to separate normal social expectations from the relationships not only permitted but demanded in intimate patient care.

It is not only in the physical sphere that the relationship may be unusual, a ward will contain a wide range of individuals of different educational backgrounds who are employed in a wide range of occupations and belong to different social classes. There will also be a wide range of individual differences between patients in terms of personality type, personal preferences, values, beliefs and perceptions. However, as far as the nurse is concerned these factors must make no difference to the way in which they are treated or receive care.

In a small community it is possible that a patient may be already known by the nurse, either personally or because of the position they hold in the community. If this is so, it is vital that the nurse should be able to detach herself from this personal knowledge to ensure impartiality. Equally, any knowledge gained during the professional relationship must not be used outside the professional interaction.

Community nurses have an additional privilege in that they are able to enter the home of their patients/clients. Once again, this will provide knowledge about the home that would not normally be available except to chosen friends. Sometimes the patient's way of life will be such that the nurse may dislike or even disapprove of it; however, unless it has bearing on the health of the patient comment should not be made nor should the details be related to other people.

The occupational health nurse has another concern: while her responsibility is the health and/or safety of the worker, management may be anxious to receive information about the worker for organisational reasons. It may be difficult in certain circumstances to separate the information which is of a privileged nature and therefore confidential from that which can legitimately be used by management. The decision has to be made on the basis of whether or not it would have been given in any situation other than that of nurse.

Often when the relationship between the patient/client and the nurse is prolonged, a friendship over and above that of a professional relationship may develop. It is in this situation that the greatest care has to be taken to avoid abusing the relationship. It is important, here, to consider the *power* relationship that exists between nurse and patient. In almost all such relationships, the nurse is necessarily in a dominant relationship vis-à-vis the patient, often due to the fact that the patient is always dependent upon the nurse: it is never a case of the nurse being dependent upon the patient. Thus, the relationship is unequal.

This unequal relationship may echo the earlier parent/child relationship and may be similar to what is known in psychotherapy as 'transference' (Procter 1978; Schafer 1983). When transference occurs in the nursing relationship, the patient comes to view the nurse as having all those positive qualities that she, the patient, once saw in her mother or father. (This is 'positive' transference. In 'negative' transference, the patient sees in the nurse all sorts of negative parental qualities. Fortunately in nursing, this negative transference is likely to be less common!) This unconscious mental process may lead to the patient becoming very dependent upon the nurse; examples of this may be when the patient suggests that a particular nurse is 'his' nurse, or is 'more understanding' than other nurses. Such compliments may be very flattering and are, of course, genuinely felt by the patient. All nurses need to be aware that this deeper level of dependence may occur and that it may bring with it the desire of the patient to ask for a closer relationship with that nurse.

It is particularly important for the longer-term nurse/patient relationship to be 'ended' gently and slowly by the nurse concerned. The process of 'saying goodbye' should be considered as soon as the nurse realises that an end to the relationship is in sight. Very often the patient who has become very dependent will deny that the end of the relationship is going to occur at all. In this case, the patient continues to act as though the relationship will carry on indefinitely and may be very hurt when ultimately it comes to an end. It is easy for the nurse to underestimate how much a nurse/patient relationship can mean to the patient. It is vital, however, that the nurse should differentiate between a professional relationship and a friendship. Whilst it is tempting to think that there need be no difference between the two and that patients can be 'friends', such a position fails to acknowledge the complex set of psychological processes that may be occurring when a dependent, often sick, person is meeting a 'caregiver'. The relationship that develops out of this set of circumstances is usually very different from the circumstances that surround the more usual development of a friendship. In an ordinary friendship, the two people involved are usually of relatively equal status and are free to choose whether or not they become emotionally attached to each other. In the nurse/patient relationship, as we have seen, the two people involved do not informally 'choose' each other but find themselves together in a complex web of emotional, physical and social circumstances.

In psychiatric nursing, the need to appreciate the boundaries of relationships is, perhaps, even more acute. The nature of the psychiatric nurse/patient relationship is such that the patient will often disclose to the nurse a considerable amount of his personal feelings and such disclosure can lead to dependence. It is important that the psychiatric nurse has a strong sense of her 'ego boundary' – of the difference between her own identity and the identity of the patient. Thus, a degree of self-awareness is required here: through understanding something of our own make-up, we learn to discriminate between ourself and the other person (Bond 1986; Burnard 1985). Without such awareness there is a danger of blurring the distinction between our personal feelings and the feelings of the patient. Such blurring of roles and identities leads to confusion on the part of the patient and can lead to emotional exhaustion on the part of the nurse.

In the past, nurses were encouraged *never* to become emotionally involved with patients. In recent years the notion of being able to be totally objective in relationships has been called into question: perhaps, in the end, it is a question of balance and of being able to judge the issue of 'therapeutic distance'. On the one hand, if the nurse distances herself from the patient, she will be unable to empathise. In this case, she stands in what Martin Buber (1958) called an 'I – it' relationship to the patient: the patient is in danger of becoming an 'object', or a 'thing'. A classic example of how patients may be turned into things through this distancing is seen whenever one is referred to by diagnosis – 'The appendix in bed 6'. If, however, she stands too close, she will be so involved that she will find it difficult to sort out her own emotions from those of the patient. The skill lies in establishing the optimum point in which to stand in relation to the patient – neither too detached, nor too involved: a relationsip that Buber called the 'I – thou' relationship and one in which both parties meet as human beings. A counsel of perfection, perhaps! In everyday life, such emotional distances are extremely hard to judge but the onus should be on the nurse to endeavour to make such judgement.

Sometimes, of course, friendships between nurses and patients *do* extend beyond the initial nurse/patient relationship. The point here is not that such relationships should *never* occur, but that the nurse has particular responsibility in considering the power balance in the relationship and should weigh very carefully whether or not a friendship that develops out of such a nurse/patient relationship is one freely chosen by the patient. It may seem strange to question whether or not friendships are 'chosen' in this way but it may be even stranger to call a state of dependence, a friendship! Just as a psychotherapist would be acting unethically if she took advantage of the strong emotions aroused in her client by the close relationship engendered by psychotherapy, so the nurse should not exploit the often equally strong emotions invoked by the administration of care.

Some situations produce particular problems, as when a patient or client is of particular interest to the press. It is obvious that journalists have a job to do and equally obvious that they have a readership avid for details of the personal lives of celebrities. In order to meet this need for information they often ask what appear to be innocuous questions which may be acutely embarrassing when used out of context. In order to avoid this problem most health authorities have a press officer and it is important that it is only that person who speaks to media representatives.

One of the first things that any nurse needs to learn is that apparently harmless gossip about who is in the ward or who has been into a clinic may be inappropriate and, in particular, such chat in a public place such as a bus or train can be overheard and possibly misused.

From this discussion it can be seen that the nurse is in a very privileged position, interacting with a wide variety of people, allowed access to information and buildings, and made privy to intimate details relating to individuals and families. This privilege carries with it the responsibility not to abuse this unique position.

REFERENCES

Bond, M. (1986) *Stress and Self-Awareness: a Guide for Nurses*. Heinemann: London.
Buber, M. (1958) *I and Thou*. Scribner: New York.
Burnard, P. (1985) *Learning Human Skills: a Guide for Nurses*. Heinemann: London.
Proctor, B. (1978) *The Counselling Shop*. Deutsch: London.
Schafer, R. (1983) *The Analytical Attitude*. Basic Books: New York.

CHAPTER 9

Confidentiality

*Respect confidential information obtained in the course
of professional practice and refrain from disclosing such
information without the consent of the patient/client, or a
person entitled to act on his/her behalf, except when
disclosure is required by law or by the order of a court or is
necessary in the public interest.*

Clause 9 of the Code of Professional Conduct emphasises that confidential information obtained in the course of professional practice should not be disclosed without the consent of the patient, or someone authorised to act on the patient's behalf, with three exceptions: the requirements of the law; by order of a court or in the public interest. Such a statement would appear to state self-evident facts; however, the issue of confidentiality raises many questions, so many in fact that the UKCC issued an elaboration of Clause 9 in an effort to clarify some of the queries raised.

The need for confidentiality is one that was recognised as far back as the compilation of the Hippocratic Oath, by which newly-qualified doctors are asked to declare:

> Whatsoever things I see or hear concerning the life of men, in my attendance on the sick or even apart therefrom, which ought not to be noised abroad, I will keep silence thereon, counting such things as sacred secrets.

As the UKCC's document explains, the focal word in the definition of confidentiality is 'trust' and without this trust no therapeutic relationship can be developed or maintained between the health care worker and the patient/client.

The level of trust placed by the patient/client in the doctor or nurse is very high indeed. It results in the disclosure of personal details, the submission to intimate examination, both physical and mental, and the agreement to, and co-operation in, often unpleasant treatment regimens. In return for this trust the patient/client has the right to expect that information given and details of mind and body revealed will be respected and only used in a therapeutic manner.

This is an interesting example of the fact that *rights and duties* are, in effect, opposite sides of the same coin. In the doctor or nurse patient/client relationship the pattern is as shown in Figure 9.1.

Doctor/nurse		Patient/client	
Right	*Duty*	*Right*	*Duty*
Information	Confidentiality	Knowledge	Reveal data
Access to mental/ physical data	Treatment	Confidentiality	Co-operation

Figure 9.1

By agreeing to enter into a relationship with healtn care professionals the patient/client tacitly agrees to divulge appropriate information to them; however, one of the potential problems relating to the maintenance of confidentiality is that in most cases the person is not cared for by one individual but by a team made up of a wide variety of workers. In this situation it is essential that all the team members have access to the relevant information and patients/ clients are generally aware of this fact and therefore their consent to the availability of data is implied.

One problem is to decide who the team members really are and hence who should have access to records. It may be clearly understood by a patient that the doctor and nurse need information and probably few would question the physotherapist's right of access to the patient's file, but has the hospital chaplain the same right of access, and what should be the position of the wide range of students who may be involved in the organisation?

The patient/client may regard some personal information as being of such a sensitive nature that a request is made that access to it be restricted. This request should be honoured and if subsequently it becomes apparent that an individual, not originally considered to need the information, is found to require it for the good of the patient/client, then specific permission to the sharing of the knowledge must be obtained. This can cause difficulties in some cases: for instance, a patient may confide in a nurse and request that no other person be told yet the nurse may recognise that this information is needed by the doctor if appropriate action is to be taken. In this case the nurse should not divulge the information but explain to the patient/client why it is vital for the doctor to be told and the disadvantage that secrecy will cause.

Even more difficult is the situation that occurs when a nurse or doctor is told, or finds out by accident, details which may not directly affect the patient/client's care but have major implications for the rest of society. An example of such information may be evidence of criminal activity, such as trafficking in drugs or child abuse.

The Code itself highlights this potential difficulty in that the opening paragraph talks about 'acting at all times in the interests of society' yet emphasises that 'above all the interest of individual patient and clients must be safeguarded'. However, Clause 9 does allow for disclosure in exceptional cases, '. . .when the law requires it, when the court orders it or when it is necessary in the public interest.'

The UKCC's leaflet, in discussing this dilemma, recognises the strain that this situation may place on the individual practitioner who has to decide when disclosure is not only permissible but necessary. The recommendation is that the practitioner should seek advice from other practitioners, not only from nurses, midwives and health visitors, but also from other professionals and, in addition, it may be both wise and helpful to consult with the appropriate professional organisation. The implications of the disclosure of information must be considered from all angles before the final decision is reached.

While the discussion so far has focused on the professional's responsibility to maintain confidentiality, the DHSS Working Group on Confidentiality has suggested that employment contracts of those who handle confidential records, for example medical secretaries and record clerks, should contain the following clause:

> In the course of your duties you may have access to confidential material

about patients, members of staff or other health service business. On no account must information relating to identifiable patients be divulged to anyone other than authorised persons, for example medical, nursing or other professional staff, as appropriate, who are concerned directly with the care, diagnosis and/or treatment of the patient. If you are in any doubt whatsoever as to the authority of a person or body asking for information of this nature you must seek advice from your superior officer. Similarly, no information of a personal or confidential nature concerning individual members of staff should be divulged to anyone without the proper authority having first been given. Failure to observe these rules will be regarded by your employers as serious misconduct which could result in serious disciplinary action being taken against you, including dismissal.

The fact that confidential information is contained in personal records has been a contentious issue for many years. Many patients/clients have been suspicious about what has been recorded, especially as traditional wisdom and many health agency policies deny them the right to see these records. The Data Protection Act 1984 legally protects 'automatically processed information' which, in practice, normally means computerised records. Under this Act, any material kept on a computor record for 40 days or more must be made available for inspection. However, the Act does not cover data processed manually. Data users, that is, individuals who control the contents and use of personal data which is automatically processed, must register the type of data that they hold, how it is obtained and the purpose for which it is required.

The medical profession has been very disturbed by the requirements of this Act, asserting that access by the patient to medical notes might be harmful, break down the trust between the patient/client and the doctor, or inhibit the keeping of full and frank records. In 1986 the British Medical Association voted to urge the Health Minister to exempt medical records from the Data Protection Act: however, at the time of writing this has not been done.

The fact that some records are recorded manually and others automatically may produce an unacceptable anomaly in the patient/client's right of access to information and it would appear sensible for the same conditions to apply to all records. However, it is important to stress that the right of access is held by the individual patient or client and not by relatives (unless in a guardianship role).

The UKCC's document on confidentiality summarises the principles on which professional judgement should be based in the following manner:

1. That a patient/client has a right to expect that information given in confidence will be used only for the purpose for which it was given and will not be released to others without the patient's consent.
2. That practitioners recognise the fundamental right of their patients/clients to have information about them held in secure and private storage.
3. That where it is deemed appropriate to share information obtained in the course of professional practice with other health or social work practitioners, the practitioner who obtained the information must ensure, as far as it is reasonable, before its release that it is being imparted in strict professional confidence and for a specific purpose.
4. That, the responsibility either to disclose or withhold confidential information in the public interest lies with the individual practitioner, that he or she cannot delegate the decision, and that he or she cannot be required by a superior to disclose or withhold information against his or her will.
5. That a practitioner who chooses to breach the basic principle of confidentiality in the belief that it is necessary in the public interest must have considered the matter sufficiently to justify that decision.
6. That deliberate breaches of confidentiality other than with the consent of the patient/client should be exceptional.

REFERENCES

Code of Professional Conduct (1984) UKCC: London.
Confidentiality – A UKCC Advisory Paper (1987) UKCC: London.
Data Protection Act (1984) HMSO: London
Report of the Confidentiality Working Group of the DHSS Steering Group on Health Service Information: London.

CHAPTER 10

Caring for Others

Have regard to the environment of care and its physical, psychological and social effects on patients/clients, and also to the adequacy of resources, and make known to appropriate persons or authorities any circumstances which could place patients/clients in jeopardy of which militate against safe standards of practice.

The tenth statement of the Code of Conduct contains a considerable number of important points, some of which have been alluded to in other chapters. It is worth considering each of them in turn.

First is the notion of the environment of care. What may be said to make up such an environment? One factor which may decide this is *where* the caring takes place. In a simple sense, the likelihood is that it will either take place in a hospital ward or department or that it will take place in the patient's home. If the environment of care is a clinical department of a hospital, that environment will contain not only the fixtures and fittings of the ward but also the whole 'climate' of the hospital – the attitudes of the staff, the interpersonal skills demonstrated by such staff and a whole range of almost subliminal things that bombard the patient as consumer of care. Clearly, then, the nurse has some responsibility to consider her part in creating an environment of care which is, indeed, *caring*. Care does not stop at offering a range of clinical procedures but includes the whole atmosphere that surrounds the patient during his stay.

In a similar but different sense, the environment of care, when it is the patient's home, will also affect that patient's health. Whilst the surroundings may be familiar to the patient, it is likely that they will be *perceived* in a different way when that person becomes a patient in his own home. Once a person is designated as 'ill' by another family member, that person tends to be viewed differently by the rest of the family and thus will come to view their home circumstances differently. In this sense, then, the 'environment of care' includes the family itself. Again, the nurse needs to take this fact into account when caring for the patient at home.

This leads to the second set of concepts contained in this statement within the Code of Conduct. It asks that the nurse should consider the physical, psychological and social effects of the environment on the patient. Most nurses will be familiar with the sort of physical considerations that must be borne in mind regarding how the environment affects the patient. A short list of such considerations would include such matters as heating, lighting, ventilation, freedom from pain, adequate diet, sleep and attention to body functions. There are, of course, many other considerations and the reader is referred to Hunt and Sendell (1983), Du Gas (1983) and Faulkner (1985) for more detailed discussions of the physical considerations of patient care. In a sense, the main *ethical* consideration here is that physical care is carried out thoroughly and with due attention. In some hospitals, this will be further clarified by recourse to a procedure manual of some kind; in others, it will be through discussion of a range of principles of physical care.

The psychological effects of the climate of care are more nebulous and less easy to spell out. We all view the world from a different perspective. How each of us views the experience of illness will vary from person to person. The danger must always be in our *generalising* about a person's psychological make-up or their psychological reaction to their environment. George Kelly (1955), the personal construct psychologist, noted that if you want to know how someone feels, ask them, they might just tell you! This may give us a useful clue as to how to assess people's experiences of what is happening to them – we ask them and continue to check with them on how they are thinking and feeling. This would seem to be a far more appropriate method than *assuming* how a person is experiencing the world.

This approach may also give us clues as to how to use psychological research and research generated within the field of nursing. It can never be the case that research findings apply to all people in similar situations to those studied in a particular research project. All that research can do is offer us a series of *pointers* as to *what may be the case*. Thus, we must use research wisely and test out whether or not it applies to this person in this set of circumstances. It may, it may not.

The same limitation must also apply to the social effects of the caring environment on the patient. For some people, ill health is merely a brief hiccup in their life: for others, any bout of illness is of major concern. Our task as nurses is not to make value-judgements about how the patient and his family deal with illness but to *note* how they do it and act accordingly. This, again, refers back to the notion of sustained awareness that has been alluded to in other chapters in this book. It is only by constantly observing what patients are telling us that we can make decisions about how to help them. It is notable, too, that all sorts of cultural consideration will prevail here. People from different countries and cultures view and experience illness in different sorts of ways. Nurses would do well to note these cultural differences and, again, not assume that all people experience illness in the same sort of way.

The next issue dealt with in this section is having regard to the adequacy of resources. There are, in fact, at least two issues, here: one is whether or not the patient is receiving the care that he needs, and the second is whether or not resources *are available* to ensure adequate care. In order to cope with both sides of the equation it is necessary to have a firm sense both of what *is* available and what *is not* available – it is no use our having plans for a particular style of nursing care if the resources are not available to deliver it. On the other hand, it is a pity if we do not deliver the care that we could, because we are unaware of the availability of certain resources. In the end, this may be a question of knowledge. We have a duty to make ourselves conversant with the facilities, agencies and policies of the health care environment in which we work

Linked with this concept of resources is the issue of making known to appropriate persons or authorities any circumstances which could place patients in jeopardy or which militate against safe standards of practice – the final aspect of this statement in the code. There are a number of issues involved in this notion. First, we must be clear who the 'appropriate persons or authorities' are. Usually, these are spelt out in a grievance procedure or can be obtained from senior nurses or administrators. Second, we need to know the sort of circumstances which may place patients in jeopardy or militate against safe standards of practice. Again, here, a certain level of knowledge is required. We cannot *observe* unsafe circumstances if we do not have the 'equipment' for making such observations. In this sense, the 'equipment' required is a fund of knowledge from which to draw conclusions. The very least we must have is a sense of our own limitations – of knowing when to ask for an opinion or advice from a more senior colleague. Making decisions about levels of safety can never be an abitrary affair: a situation is either safe or it is not. Sometimes such levels of safety are spelt out in a document issued by a particular health authority under the Health and Safety at Work Act 1974. In other cases such levels are passed on through 'custom and practice'. In either case, it is necessary for the nurse to make an *informed* decision based on nursing and medical knowledge, appreciation of the facts of the situation at the time and on awareness of current health and safety standards.

A certain *political* awareness is also required. We need to be able to formulate questions about *why* certain standards of conduct and safety exist and *how* they came to exist. The temptation is to believe that all such standards arise out of rational decisions based on current research and theory! In an ideal world this would probably be the case, but in reality such decisions are made on much more shaky foundations, including political expediency, tradition, changing ideologies of health care, consumer expectation and even on the basis of crisis management! On many occasions, decisions about standards are made *after* an incident has occurred – what may be termed retrospective policy provision. Some of the political issues involved, here, are dealt with by Salvage (1985) and Clay (1987).

REFERENCES

Clay, T. (1987) *Nurses, Power and Politics*. Heinemann: London.
Du Gas, B.W. (1983) *Introduction to Patient Care: A Comprehensive Approach to Nursing*. W.B. Saunders: Philadelphia, PA.
Faulkner, A. (1985) *Nursing: a creative approach*. Baillière Tindall: London.
Kelly, G. (1955) *The Psychology of Personal Constructs*: Vols 1 and 2. Norton: New York.
Hunt, P. and Sendell, B. (1983) *Nursing the Adult with a Specific Physiological Disturbance*. Macmillan: Basingstoke.
Salvage, J. (1985) *The Politics of Nursing*. Heinemann: London.

CHAPTER 11

Caring for Colleagues

Have regard to the workload of and the pressures on
professional colleagues and subordinates and take
appropriate action if these are seen to be such as to constitute
abuse of the individual practitioner and/or to jeopardise safe
standards of practice.

In Chapter 5 the role of the various members of the health care team
and their relationship as team members were discussed. In this
chapter a somewhat different aspect of working together is
considered – that of mutual responsibility. It is tempting, when all
team members have their own areas of responsibility, to let each one
get on with his own task and assume that each is capable not only
of the type of work that he is assigned, but that all can work at the
same speed and withstand the same pressures. This is obviously not
necessarily the case.

It is ironic that while nurses are expected to regard each individual
patient as an unique human being entitled to individualised care,
they are often regarded as a grade or type and treated as a group
rather than as individuals. This situation exists in all areas of work:
in the ward area nurses are often described as 'second-years' or
'learners' as if such a title explained everything about them, their
level of skill, learning needs, and so on. The implication is that there
is, somewhere, a template against which each nurse is placed so that
each one is identical.

A similar situation exists in nursing education: teaching programmes are formulated in such a way that each learner is expected
to learn at the same pace. Rarely is account taken of the fact that
individuals start at different levels of knowledge, maturity and life

experience. Instead, each must conform to a set pattern of teaching methods and clinical experience, produce almost identical pieces of work for assessment purposes and in every way behave in a predetermined manner so that the result is more like the output of a jelly baby factory rather than the development of an educated professional, able to respond to whatever needs the patient and/or the service may require.

No doubt because of this expectation of 'sameness' that is created by the training programme, the same expectation extends throughout the service. Each grade has an area of built-in expectations and standards and anyone who does not fit into the mould is considered to be either slacking, incompetent, a troublemaker, or all three.

A moment's thought will demonstrate how unreasonable such an approach is: physically and psychologically each individual has strengths and weaknesses and, therefore, even if two nurses have undergone identical training programmes it is highly unlikely that they will respond to work pressures in the same way. Link with that their different life experiences, both past and present, their different aims in the profession and in life generally, and it will be seen that it is more than probable that each will view her apparent workload differently and react in an idiosyncratic manner to each situation.

Since the advent of a systematic and individualised approach to patient care it is surprising that members of health care teams have not begun to realise that as team members they are also entitled to, and should also give each other, individual care and consideration. Naturally, such an approach is not easy. It is always tempting to feel, 'If I can cope, so should they.' Item 11 of the Code states that each nurse should 'Have regard to the workload of and the pressures on professional colleagues and subordinates and take appropriate action if these are seen to be such as to constitute abuse of the individual practitioner and/or to jeopardise safe standards of practice.'

There are many examples of situations where this care may be needed. One common case is the distress that may occur on the death of a patient. Conventional nursing wisdom states that professionals do not allow themselves to become involved with the patient and therefore should not be upset when a patient dies. Despite this traditional expectation nurses have always felt grief at the death of a patient, and in situations where the patient is seen as an individual and not just as a diagnostic category some grief is inevitable and should not be denied. Distress will, however, vary with the individual and it is important that support should be provided by others in the team to those most in need. This may be simple – making a cup of coffee – or more sophisticated – as in the provision of counselling or a formalised support group. It is not only nurses who require this understanding and support, the apparently all-powerful doctor may be equally distressed, as may the ward maid, yet these people are rarely considered to need help.

A special example of the need for this type may occur when nurses are involved in caring for the victims of a major disaster. Fawcett (1987) the Sister in the Accident and Emergency Unit that received the victims of the mass shooting in Hungerford, Avon, in 1987, describes vividly the fact that during the emergency all the staff worked at a high rate and appeared to be able to cope with the demands being placed upon them; however, after the event many demonstrated both psychological and physical disturbance: 'I found my normal emotional resilience had disappeared, and this was made worse by the constant replaying of events in my mind, coupled with insomnia.' In this case support was provided by trained counsellors.

Levels of work may be such as to constitute an impossible load on staff. Nurse are renowned for 'coping' and often see it as a demonstration of failure not to be able to 'get through the work'. Such a situation is often dangerous to those being cared for, because in order to fulfil the demands of the workload shortcuts are taken and, as a result, mistakes made. In addition, individuals are often called upon to function at a level for which they have not been prepared and therefore may not be aware of what is safe practice. The misuse and abuse of the enrolled nurse, who is frequently required to function as a first-level nurse, is an example of this latter point. This is an area where nurse managers at all levels have a responsibility to ensure that if adequate levels of staffing cannot be provided then the clinical area should be reduced or closed. It is very sad to be present at a Professional Conduct Committee and to hear of a nurse who, despite the fact that representation had been made to management, had been left to cope in an impossible situation with the result that a mistake occurred resulting in damage to and sometimes the death of a patient.

It is worth considering at this point the *manner* in which the whole issue of overwork is broached by the person who experiences it, to the manager. Certain social skills are required in order to approach a manager over such an issue and considerable forethought needs to have gone into the presentation. What is required is *not* that the nurse makes an emotional and, perhaps, angry appeal to the manager but that she prepares a rational and well-thought-out set of arguments as to why she considers herself to be putting herself or her patients in jeopardy. It is often useful, too, if a series of possible solutions are identified for discussion with the manager concerned. Very few people like problems thrust upon them without either prior notice or some ideas for solutions!

Coping with a very heavy workload can be difficult in any circumstances, whether clinical, educational or management. Gortner (1977) offers some principles by which nurses may learn to cope in organisations and manage heavy and stressful workloads. These may be identified as follows:

Become competent in what you do. The person who develops the necessary skills and knowledge to work effectively and efficiently may experience subjectively less stress than the person who does not.

Know well the organisation in which you work. It is particularly valuable to become very familiar with the aims of the organisation, the power structure, the hierarchy and the lines of communication. Knowledge of these things allows the nurse to effectively *use* them to her own and others' advantage.

Be a master of the possible. It is useful to identify ways in which aspects of work and/or the organisation *can* be changed by the individual nurse. Realistic aims that can be reached are usually far less frustrating than highly idealistic ones which may lead to frustration!

Recognise and seize the opportunity for doing more. On the face of it, this may seem a curious suggestion for someone who is already working very hard. On reflection, however, it may be identified that it is only through attempting new projects and developing innovative strategic plans that the individual can develop and 'grow'. There is often a great temptation for the individual to carry on doing those things which she is good at. It is also the route towards boredom and stasis.

Consider few problems to be original. Hence the solution is somewhere and that is the challenge. When faced with continuous work pressure, the temptation is to assume that 'nothing can be done' or that 'this situation is so difficult it can never be remedied'. As Gortner points out, however, few problems are *really* that new or that difficult. The act of treating them as a challenge can help in the generation of innovative solutions. *Recognise the value of support systems. Build and use some for yourself.* As we are suggesting in this chapter, colleagues and peers can often be a fruitful source of support. It is often useful if such peer support is *formalised*, and regular peer support groups are set up in which a forum is offered for the discussion of current work-related problems.

Know yourself well. A frequent theme running through the present book is that of developing self-awareness. One of the first stages in dealing with organisational or work-related stress is knowing personal limitations and areas of vulnerability. This is, indeed, a key practical and ethical issue, for as Shakespeare said: 'This above all: to thine own self be true, and it must follow, as the night the day, Thou cans't not then be false to any man...'

One of the results of continuous work overload may be burn-out (Shubin 1978; Storlie 1979). This may be defined as an evolutionary and insidious process of growing emotional exhaustion occurring as a consequence of being exposed to chronic job-related stress factors. Three degrees of burn-out may be identified. The characteristics of first-degree burn-out include short-lived bouts of irritability, fatigue and worry, and a tendency perpetually to view work situations and colleague-relationships in a pessimistic and negative light. Second-degree burn-out may be viewed as a worsening of the situation, accompanied by feelings of failure, lack of interest in work and a sense of powerlessness and inadequacy. With the onset of third-degree burn-out comes the development of psychosomatic ailments. Excessive sick leave, the overuse of alcohol and, perhaps, the excessive use of minor tranquillisers are also symptomatic. With all these changes comes a deep sense of job dissatisfaction. This is ofen manifest in a sarcastic and cynical manner and a tendency to be judgemental and overcritical of others.

A variety of factors may account for this state of burn-out. Age and the health status of the nurse are important physical factors. Social factors such as the personal relationships of the individual and the quality of the homelife of that person need to be considered. Environmental factors such as workspace, colour, brightness, noise and proximity of other colleagues all play their part. Psychological factors such as the personality of the individual and their problem-solving skills, influence the degree to which nurses avoid or develop burn-out. Ideological factors such as how authentic the individual feels in her role, the degree to which she feels fulfilled by her job and how much she feels able to invest in relationships with patients all contribute to coping or burning out. Organisational factors such as career position and the rate of organisational change all need to be taken into account.

Because of the insidious nature of burn-out or job-related stress, the individual who suffers from it may be unaware that it is happening at all. It falls upon colleagues, then, to be vigilant for signs of it in others when work pressure is particularly high. Whilst self-monitoring of stress levels is the ideal, it is often impossible for the hard-working person to notice the stress that they are suffering but which is only too noticeable to those around her! Altruism should not be reserved only for patients but should be freely applied to colleagues. Nursing is, after all, a *caring* profession.

As has already been mentioned, one of the characters in Charles Kingsley's book *The Water Babies* is Mrs Do-As-You-Would-Be-Done-By, and this could well have served as the title of this chapter. It may be at some personal cost that a colleague is supported during a period of stress; however, it is unlikely that such altruism will go unrewarded as care for each other becomes the norm. The philosopher Kant (1785) expressed the situation in his *Fundamental Principles of Morals* when trying to lay down rules of moral behaviour which he described as Categorical Imperatives, as quoted in Chapter 7:

> Act only on that maxim through which you can at the same time will that it should become an universal law.

Another aspect of this caring for others is the responsibility each person has when delegating work to another to ensure that the person to whom the task is assigned both understands what is required and is capable of carrying it out. This is particularly important when dealing with learners but applies to all aspects of delegation. This is not a one-sided responsibility: the person to whom the task is delegated also has the duty to inform the person delegating if the task is not understood or outside her field of competence. Once again, this is an area where tradition makes it difficult for some people to admit that they 'don't know how', and it is important that the unit environment is such that individuals do not feel threatened by an admission of ignorance.

Pyne (1987), writing about the formulation of the Code, says:

Many practitioners now understand that it is respectable to challenge and complain where that is necessary and to accept that to do so is an intrinsic part of proper professional behaviour. I believe that we are steadily observing a revolution in conduct as practising members of the profession accept that the previously held view of 'good conduct' as being compliant and submissive was not only wrong, but responsible for many of the problems that nursing has faced.

While agreeing with these statements, it may be necessary in some cases for a nurse to speak up for a less articulate or confident colleague to ensure that neither the individual is abused nor patients suffer.

REFERENCES

Fawcett J. (1987) Diary of a Disaster. *Nursing Times*, **83**:43.
Gortner, S.R. (1977) Strategies for Survival in the Practical World. *American Journal of Nursing*, **77**:618-619.
Kant, I. (1785) *Fundamental Principles of the Metaphysics of Morals* (trans. Abbott, T.K.). Library of Literal Arts: New York.
Pyne R. (1987) Top Secret Code. *Nursing Times*, **83**:42.
Shakespeare, W. *Hamlet*, I.iii.
Shubin, S. (1978) Burn-out: the Professional Hazard in Nursing. *Nursing*, **18**:7.
Storlie, F. (1979) Burn-out: the elaboration of a concept. *American Journal of Nursing*, **79**.

CHAPTER 12

Assisting the
Development of Colleagues

*In the context of the individual's own knowledge,
experience and sphere of authority, assist peers and
subordinates to develop professional competence in accordance
with their needs.*

In considering how to assist peers and subordinates to develop professional competence it may be worth examining how we can identify or give shape to our own knowledge and experience. After all, as the statement above notes, it is from those domains (alongside our sphere of authority) that we draw the necessary skills to help others.

A practical method of dividing up knowledge and experience in order to understand it is to consider the following three domains: propositional knowledge, practical knowledge and experiential knowledge (Heron 1981; Burnard 1987). Propositional knowlege is 'textbook' knowledge – theories, facts, models and other theoretical constructions. We need such propositional knowledge in order that we may make sense of the world around us. Theories and models help us to classify things and to categorise them in such a way as to make them intelligible. They can also help us to plan for the future, for an accurate theory usually enables us to *predict*, with varying degrees of accuracy what will happen next.

Practical knowledge is knowledge gained through doing. Every time we give an injection skillfully we display practical knowledge. Practical knowledge often involves psychomotor activity and manual dexterity, but it may not. An example of the demonstration of practical knowledge which does not involve psychomotor activity is the display of counselling skills. Such skills may be developed systematically through attendance on a counselling course or through the process of *doing* counselling. Either way, the skilled nurse-as-counsellor exhibits distinct practical knowledge every time she successfully counsels someone.

There are important differences between propositional knowledge and practical knowledge. Propositional knowledge involves what Ryle (1949) called 'knowing that' something is the case. Thus, I may know that certain things are important in order for me to deliver a baby without actually posessing the skills to do so! Practical knowledge, on the other hand, involves what Ryle called 'knowing how'. Thus, I may know how to deliver a baby and be able to carry through the process without knowing the theoretical implications of what I am doing. Clearly, it is better that we combine both propositional and practical knowledge. What we know in a theoretical sense should tie up precisely with what we do in practice.

Experiential knowledge, on the other hand, is personal knowledge through direct encounter with a person, place or thing. Thus, before I went to America, I had a considerable amount of propositional knowledge about the place: I had pictures in my mind about how certain places looked and I knew something of the history of America. When I visited the country, however, everything I 'knew' about it previously was changed by my direct encounter with it. This, then, is experiential knowledge. Experiential knowledge is knowledge that is personal to the individual. It is gained, as is suggested by the name, through personal experience. We cannot give another person experiential knowledge nor can we teach it to others. In recent years there has been increasing interest in the use of experiential learning methods (Kagan 1985; Kagan et al. 1986; Burnard 1985) in nurse education. These methods are concerned precisely with the development of experiential knowledge: understanding the world through direct encounter with it. In another sense, too, much nursing skill is learned not through the school or college of nursing but by direct experience: we learn nursing by doing it.

However, there are limits to the value of experiential knowledge just as there are limits to the value of propositional and practical knowledge. We cannot wisely rely *only* on our personal experience. To do this would be to limit our knowledge base in a very important sense: if we rely only on our own experience we never give attention to the thinking or practice that have been developed by countless other people in the profession. Nor do we heed the research that has been conducted in the field. What we may choose to do, however, is to test the theories, skills and research of others for ourselves and thus combine the domains of propostional, practical and experiential knowledge.

Consideration of the above three domains of knowledge may help us to assess our own knowledge levels. When we consider our knowledge of nursing, for example, are we clear about our theoretical deficits and assets (propositional knowledge)? Can we readily identify the skills that we have and those we lack (practical knowledge)? Are we able reflectively to consider our past experience and be clear about the experience we need in the future (experiential knowledge)? If we can do all these things then we are in a stronger postion for helping others to develop professional competence. Without that self-assessment we are blind to our own deficiencies and competencies. That blindness may further blind us to the deficiencies and competencies of others.

Note that it is not being suggested that we have to *rectify* all our deficiencies before we help others. All we have to do is to identify them, to know that they are there. Armed with this knowledge, we can be better equipped to notice the theoretical, practical and experiential gaps in others. Whether or not we then go on to plug our own knowledge gaps is another ethical issue! It would seem difficult to justify on any grounds that having acknowledged our ignorance or lack of expertise or experience in a particular field, we then do nothing about it. A variant of the 'golden rule' may apply here. The golden rule is that we should do unto others only that which we would have done to us. The variant, here, may be that we should only advise others about their knowledge base if we are prepared to do something about our own.

Once we are clear, then, about our own sphere of knowledge and experience we are better able to assist others. We need, also, to be clear about our 'sphere of authority', as referred to in the Code of Conduct. For most practical purposes, our sphere of authority is set out formally in our job description. In another sense, though, that authority is granted less formally through the process of 'custom and practice'. We gain authority to carry out certain tasks through actually doing them: the more we continue to do them, the more they become legitimated. It would seem wise for us to take stock regularly of what it is we do in our jobs and compare what we *actually* do with what we are *required* to do. This, again, calls for the vigilant sense of awareness called for in previous chapters.

In helping others to develop, it is essential, first of all, that we should *listen* to them and try to enter their 'frame of reference' − their view of the world. The great temptation is to imagine that everyone views the world as we do. The truth is, of course, that we all view the same or similar situations quite differently. Such perceptual differences may be accounted for by the fact of our differences of physiology, background, upbringing, culture, education and personality. We have also lived unique lives and experienced the world as no other person. Given these individual differences, it is vital that we learn to listen to the other person carefully, for it is only through such intense listening that we can hope to enter into the frame of reference of the other person.

Many courses that offer basic counselling skills are now available in colleges and extramural departments. Almost all such courses emphasise this need for accurate listening and offer exercises for the development of the art and skill of listening. Basic listening and attending skills are also being introduced into nurse training programmes. In psychiatric nursing, such skills are seen as essential and prescribed by the 1982 Syllabus of Training (ENB 1982). Whether through basic nurse training or through attendance at a course of training, it is recommended that all nurses undergo some sort of listening skills training.

If such formal training is not available, individuals can do much to sharpen up their skills on their own. One very simple exercise is merely to sit with a friend or colleague and pay full attention to what she is saying. This involves temporarily 'suspending judgement' or being critical of what she is saying: the aim is purely to hear what she says. Such an exercise constitues part of what Heron (1973) calls 'conscious use of self'. By this is meant the constant *choosing* of a particular type of behaviour (in this case, listening) rather than merely letting our behaviour 'happen'. We *can* train ourselves to be more effective listeners and the conscious effort involved can mean that we understand others more clearly.

Once we have heard the other person, we can help her assess her own needs in terms of professional competence. It is worth noting the emphasis made by the Code of Conduct: we are requested to assist peers '. . . in accordance with *their* needs'. Note that it is not *my perception* of their needs − the needs are to be defined by the person concerned. Thus we need to develop skills in helping others to identify their own needs. This can be done through the process of listening described above, and through the use of questions that encourage the other person to problem-solve. Such questions can be aimed at encouraging the other person to identify gaps in her knowledge or skill. Examples of such questions may be:

'What do you need to learn next?'
'What sort of information may help you now?'
'Can you identify the nursing procedure that you carry out effectively and those that your not so sure about?'
Or simply:
'What do you need to do next?'

In each of the above cases, it is the individual herself who is responsible for identifying areas for further development, whether in the domains of propositional, practical or experiential knowledge. Such an approach is quite in keeping with progressive approaches to education and training which stress a student-centred approach (Knowles 1978; 1981; Rogers 1983). If we are to encourage our patients to develop autonomy and to take part in planning part of their care, it is reasonable that nurses develop their own skill and knowledge levels through this student-centred approach.

REFERENCES

Burnard, P. (1985) *Learning Human Skills: a guide for nurses.* Heinemann: London.

Burnard, P. (1987) Towards an epistemological basis for experiential learning in nurse education. *Journal of Advanced Nursing,* **12**:189-193.

ENB (1982) *Syllabus of Training: Professional Register,* Part 3 (Registered Mental Nurse). English and Welsh National Boards for Nursing, Midwifery and Health Visiting, London and Cardiff.

Heron, J. (1973) *Experiential Training Techniques.* Human Potential Research Project, University of Surrey: Guildford.

Heron, J. (1981) Philosophical basis for a new paradigm. In Reason, P. and Rowan, J. *Human Inquiry: a sourcebook of new paradigm research.* Wiley: Chichester.

Kagan, C. (ed.) (1985) *Interpersonal Skills in Nursing: Research and Applications*: Croom Helm: London.

Kagan, C, Evans, J. and Kay, B. (1986) *A Manual of Interspersonal Skills for Nurses: an Experiential Approach,* Harper and Row: London.

Knowles, M (1978) *The Adult Learner: a neglected species.* Gulf: Texas.

Knowles, M. (1981) *The Modern Practice of Adult Education.* Follett: Chicago.

Rogers, C.R. (1983) *Freedom to Learn for the Eighties.* Merrill: Columbus, Ohio.

Ryle, G. (1949) *The Concept of Mind.* Peregrine: Harmondsworth.

CHAPTER 13

Rewards

*Refuse to accept any gift, favour or hospitality which might
be interpreted as seeking to exert undue influence to obtain
preferential consideration'.*

A great deal of energy is exerted in trying to find out why nurses
leave the profession, often very soon after qualifying. While the
answer to this question is obviously important, perhaps it is
suprising that any stay. Not only does the nurse work unsocial hours
and undertake hard physical work but he or she spends the day with
people who are at their least attractive due to illness pain and
distress. Nevertheless, many nurses spend all their working life in
the profession and would not consider doing anything else. Even
though rates of pay have improved in recent years they are not
sufficiently attractive to be the main reason why these nurses are
happy in their work.

All people seek satisfaction in their daily life, and this can be
provided in a number of ways. It is quite common to talk about
'meeting the patient's needs' but nurses also have needs and it is the
way in which these are or are not met that decides whether or not
they remain in the profession.

This meeting of needs is, of course, not restricted to nurses, and
social anthropologists have described it as a form of 'social
exchange'. Cynics argue that little is done in the world from purely
altruistic motives but that in every activity there is a reward of some
sort. While some aspects of social exchange have a complex
economic connotation, other aspects apear to be important for their
symbolic value and the social ties that they create. For example,
Malinowski (1922), states that there is a

> fundamental human impulse to display, to share, to bestow; the deep tendency to create social ties through the exchange of gifts . . . giving for the sake of giving is one of the most important features of Trobriand society and, from its very general and fundamental nature, I submit it is a universal feature of all primitive societies.

A more recent writer, Lévi-Strauss (1969), points out that even in western society there is a strong feeling towards reciprocity which extends to invitations, Christmas cards and birthday presents; all of which by their exchange indicate social ties between giver and recipient. Gouldner (1969) also develops this idea and states that '. . . it would seem that there can be stable patterns of reciprocity "qua" exchange only in so far as each party has both rights and duties.'

Homans (1961) considers that the process of exchange will only continue if the participants derive some benefit from it:

> The open secret of human exchange is to give to the other man behaviour that is more valuable to him than it is costly to you and to get from him behaviour that is more valuable to you than it is costly to him

The position of health care within the United Kingdom is such that it is frequently considered 'free' because payment is not made at the point of delivery. So with nursing care, many patients feel that they get more care than that which is paid for by either their insurance contributions or by the salary that the nurse receives. Thus, there is an interesting relationship where the nurse may be seen as a giver of a gift – her care – and the patient as the receiver of the gift, without the normal provision for the return of gifts. Indeed, there is no equality in the relationship of nurse and patient at the time that care is being given. Although the patient may only be in a state of temporary dependence, in the case of the chronic sick, handicapped or dying the dependence may be permanent. Therefore it may be considered that repayment for nursing care is impossible. It is this inequality of relationship that places nursing in the category of occupations which are considered vocational by the general public and which gives nurses much of their esteem. An effort to restore this balance is frequently made by the patient by the gift of gratitude.

However, in view of the reasons why individuals take up nursing it may be that they are repaid in that the dependence of the patient satisfies the nurse's psychological needs. Nurses themselves tend to indicate that this is the case and if not prevented may prolong the patient's dependency. Titmus (1970) calls this activity 'creative altruism' – creative in the sense that the self is realised with the help of others. In discussing blood donors, he says that giving blood 'allows the biological need to help to express itself'. Tonnies (Loomis 1955) sees such activity more cynically saying 'Do, ut, des' – 'What I do for you, I do only as a means to effect your simultaneous, previous or later service for me. . . . To get something from you is my end, my service is thereto which I contribute unwillingly.'

Maybe this sort of statement throws light on the fact that care of some classes of patients is seen as less prestigious in the eyes of society, which tends to classify the worth of individuals in relation to the contribution that they are able to make to society. It is not difficult to see that the stigma of dependency rests most heavily on the old, the chronically sick the mentally handicapped and those who are unlikely to be able to recover and make a contribution to society. This stigmatisation may also rest on those who care for these people and may account for the fact that those who consider nursing a vocation may choose to work with these groups. Pinker (1971) has described this situation, where the individual is unlikely to be able to repay, as one where the person is subject to a 'compassion gap'. Furthermore, he points out that the relationship between the giver and the receiver is always inherently an unstable and unequal one and that although gratitude may be used to help to restore the balance, because the gift was given first the gratitude may be given with a sense of coercion. Money is the commodity which produces instant equivalence. Social exchange in this context may be most easily depicted as a balance: on one side are the nurses' needs and on the other side the satisfactions provided by caring for patients/clients.

Meeting the Nurse's Needs.

Nurse's Needs	*Patient's Needs*
Knowledge	Information
To give physical care	Physical care
To develop skills	Psychological care
Have happy patients	

Obviously, different nurses have different emphases relating to these needs. Some have a great need to provide physical care, others have a great thirst for knowledge, and so on. Most meet their needs by working in the area that provides the greatest opportunity to match their needs with those of the patient. A nurse getting most satisfaction from physical care will be likely to work with long-stay, continuing-care patients. Those with a desire to increase their knowledge of medical science will seek work in acute units, possibly intensive care.

Patients rarely appreciate this situation and frequently say 'How can I repay you, nurse?', little realising that the very fact that they are in the role of patient makes it possible for the role of nurse to exist. All this would indicate that the interaction between nurse and patient must inevitably produce feelings of stigma on behalf of the patient and it is to overcome this discomfort that some patients may offer the nurse a gift, either in kind or money.

While verbal gratitude is greatly welcomed by nurses and, indeed, Stockwell (1976) found that nurses felt it was their right, the giving of gifts to express gratitude is more contentious. Many health authorities have a policy stating that individuals must not receive gifts from patients and that if a patient wishes to express gratitude in this way then the gift must be given either to the unit or to the authority via the administration. The reason for such a policy is easy to appreciate as it would be very easy for such a gift to be given as a bribe to ensure preferential treatment, and the Code is very clear in its statement that the nurse must 'Refuse to accept any gift, favour or hospitality which might be interpreted as seeking to exert undue influence to obtain preferential consideration.'

While most nurses are well aware of the dangers of accepting a gift which might be interpreted as a bribe from a patient, they are perhaps less sensitive to the gifts offered by pharmaceutical or other firms. In this they are not alone, as the medical profession frequently accepts hospitality from such a source. The question has to be asked, does the acceptance of a diary or the sponsorship of a conference from a commercial firm put me or my organisation under any sort of pressure to buy from that firm in preference to any other? If the answer is 'yes' then the offer of help in whatever form must be refused. If there is no pressure, not even a moral one, then it may be permissible to accept the offer: however, the relationship is always potentially a dangerous one.

In the present social setting when there is great competition for Health Service contracts the nurse has to be extremly careful not to get involved, even if unwittingly, in any activity which may constitute bribery or unfair practice.

REFERENCES.

Chapman C.M. (1984) *Theory of Nursing: Practical Application.* Harper & Row: London.

Gouldner A.W. (1960) The norm of reciprocity, a preliminary statement. *American Sociological Review,* **28**, 169.

Henderson V. (1962) *Basic Principles of Nursing Care.* ICN: Switzerland.

Homans G.C. (1961) *Social Behaviour in its Elementary Forms.* Harcourt, Brace and World: New York.

Lévi-Strauss C. (1969) *The Elementary Structures of Kinship.* Beacon Press: Boston.

Malinowski B. (1922) *Argonauts of the Western Pacific.* Routledge and Kegan Paul: New York.

Pinker R. (1971) *Social Theory and Social Policy.* Heinemann: London.

Stockwell F. (1976) *The Unpopular Patient.* Royal College of Nursing: London.

Titmus, R. (1970) *The Gift Relationship.* Allen & Unwin: London.

Tönnies F. (1887) (Trans. Loomis, P. 1955) *Community and Associations.* Routledge & Kegan Paul: London.

CHAPTER 14

Advertising

Avoid the use of professional qualifications in the promotion of commercial products in order not to compromise the independence of professional judgement on which patients/clients rely.

Nurses are always being asked by members of the general public, neighbours and friends for advice on health matters. This is inevitable and can be seen as part of the nurse's responsibility to society. Part of this advice may involve the nurse in offering her opinion on what medicine to take for a cough or how to feed a baby. In offering this advice it is likely that the nurse will mention a brand name. It is doubtful whether such advice could be considered as advertising. However, manufacturing firms may wish to have a nurse endorse their products in her professional capacity, either overtly appearing in an advertisement or covertly by accepting free or cheap samples of products which may then be passed on to patients or clients. It is this type of activity that is referred to in the final statement of the Code of Conduct.

Advertising is an activity in which the person who is the object of the advertisment is persuaded to act in a particular way. It may, in fact, be considered as a specific form of propaganda. There have been many studies to ascertain how propaganda works; one study by Katz and Lazarsfeld (1955) identified people who acted as 'opinion leaders'. These were those whose opinion was sought by friends, neighbours and acquaintances. In the area of public affairs these people tended to be of a higher social class than those seeking advice.

The medium used is also important, Lazarsfeld, Berelson and

Gaudet (1944) showed that personal influence was much more effective than any other from of communication in producing change. Influence, therefore, is likely to flow down from opinion leaders, by word of mouth, to the recipients.

Peake (1955) found that the effectiveness of information on attitude change was related to the importance of the outcome of the information on the individual. There are few areas of life that are more important to an individual than those which affect their health or that of their family. Therefore these studies are important when considering the role that may be played by professional health carers in formulating public opinion.

Nurses, midwives and health visitors are held in very great respect by the public, who credit them with a high degree of knowledge and also accord to them a high level of trust. In addition, they are people who are normally able to have personal contact with patients and because of this any product recommended by a nurses is likely to be purchased. This places a great responsibility upon the shoulders of the nurse and it is vital that any recommendation be based on the best possible knowledge and be unbiased.

Obviously, if a nurse has received payment in order to sponsor a specific product then he or she may well feel that product is the one that should be used and/or recommended even though in some cases another product would be more suitable. It is because of the danger of bias affecting professional judgement that the final statement asserts that a registered nurse, midwife and health visitor shall 'avoid the use of professional qualifications in the promotion of commercial products in order not to compromise the independent professional judgement on which patients/clients rely.'

Following the publication of the Code of Professional Conduct many questions were received at the United Kingdom Central Council from nurses who wished to become or remain involved in advertising. In an attempt to explain and elaborate on the intention of the Code, the UKCC issued a separate publication entitled *Advertising*. This document explains when and how the nurse, midwife and health visitor may be involved in using a professional qualification and not be guilty of professional misconduct, and which situations are to be avoided. It describes the following situations:

Advertising for professional work is allowed provided that such an advertisement is not ostentatious and does not imply that the practitioner is to be preferred over others. This advertisement may be for general work or be for work in some speciality in which case it is permissible to state the fact the the practitioner has completed a specialist course and has a recorded qualification.

A nurse, midwife or health visitor who owns or manages a business associated with professional practice (for example, a nursing home) may use the appropriate qualifications in advertisements for that business or on letterheadings, etc.

A nurse, midwife or health visitor employed by another person or business which requires him/her to call on other health care professionals or institutions to promote products may use the appropriate qualifications on visiting cards or other stationery.

Nurses, midwives and health visitors may be involved in providing advice for writing or featuring in promotional literature or films associated with commercial products. In this case, the appearance of the professional's name in the credits should not be accompanied by the qualification status. However, if the production is for educational or documentary purposes and could not be considered in any way as advertising, then the registration status may be stated. In addition, the practitioner may use registration qualifications in association with participation in conferences, and in radio or television programmes, providing that such participation cannot be seen to be a way of advertising the practitioner.

Advertising for professional work outside nursing, midwifery or health visiting, i. e. within the province of another profession, should not be undertaken if that other profession does not allow its practitioners to advertise. If the other profession does allow advertising and the registered nurse, midwife or health visitor wishes to use his/her registered qualification, advice and permission should first be obtained from the UKCC.

This guidance document (which is not quoted in full) should be consulted by any registered nurse, midwife or health visitor who is in any doubt regarding his/her proposed action. To summarise, attitude change is most likely to occur when the person presenting the information is of a higher social class of than those receiving the message, is in a position of trust, and is able to give the information verbally.

As stated elsewhere, the registered nurse practitioner has a special place in society. The possession of a registered qualification implies not only the achievement of specific skills and knowledge but also the holding of specific values and attitudes. This privileged status offered to members of the caring professions must not be abused and this may require a high standard of behaviour in all areas of life. Most professionals accept this and act accordingly; however, not all are sufficiently aware of the effect that the use of their qualifications may have when linked with commercial products. In a similar way, not all are sensitive to the restraint that may be placed upon them by the acceptance of gifts or hospitality from commercial firms.

REFERENCES

Advertising by Registered Nurses, Midwives and Health Visitors (1985) UKCC: London.

Katz D. and Lazarsfeld P.F. (1955) *Personal Influence: The part played by people in the flow of mass communication.* Free Press: Glencoe, Ill.

Lazarsfeld P.F., Berelson B. and Gaudet H. (1944) *The People's Choice.* Duell, Sloan & Pearce: New York.

Peake H. (1955) Attitude And Motivation. In Jones M.R. (ed.) *Nebraska Symposium on Motivation.* University Nebraska Press: Lincoln.

CHAPTER 15

Conclusion

In the preceding chapters we have explored a variety of theories and practical approaches to ethical and professional issues in nursing. In one sense, how we decide to act in a nursing situation is determined for us by the Code of Conduct. The Code lays down broad principles and offers a framework to guide professional action. What we as individuals have to do, however, is to *interpret* those principles, and very often we have to decide for ourselves what we are to do. Again, this book has offered some pointers as to how such decisions may be made. The book cannot *make* those decisions, nor can it account for the many and varied situations that arise in everyday nursing practice that are 'exceptions to the rule'. After all, in real life, situations are rarely experienced as they are printed in books!

In closing, it may be worth reconsidering some of the ways of making ethical and professional decisions that have been alluded to in this book. First, we may appeal to a code of conduct as a means of decision-making. Clearly, as this book is about such a code, it is felt that codes can be a useful means of helping and guiding the decision-making process. There are, of course, other codes that can be referred to, the most notable being particular ethical codes as outlined within specific religious sects. We have noted, too, that atheists and agnostics may also have personal codes to which they refer.

Another means of making ethical and professional decisions is through considerations of conscience. Freud called a person's conscience his 'superego' and argued that the development of such a conscience or superego evolved out of the internalisation of parental values, beliefs and attitudes at an early age (Hall 1954). Thus, when we appeal to our conscience it is as though we were experiencing one or both of our parents 'looking over our shoulder' as we make a particular decision. Another way of viewing the development of conscience is to see it in terms of socialisation. As a person grows and develops, he absorbs and learns the particular set of beliefs and values of his parents and also takes account of the broader set of beliefs and values of the particular culture in which he grows up. This process of socialisation must clearly affect decision-making. Decisions are not made in isolation nor are they made outside the particular culture in which the decision-maker lives.

This notion of culture-bound, ethical and professional decisions is an important one. It is tempting to believe that the beliefs and values of 'our' culture are the 'right' ones. Clearly, different cultures produce different values and different values will be reflected in different sorts of ethical and professional decisions, made in different countries and societies.

Another approach to ethical and professional decision-making is via the notion of utilitarianism, which argues that what is good and right is that which creates the greatest happiness for the greatest number. Indeed, many decisions are made on this basis but we may want to ponder on (a) who decides what is likely to create the greatest good, and (b) what happens to those that are not contained within the 'greatest number'.

It may be worth considering, too, Sartre's (1956; 1973) notion of 'situational ethics'. In order to understand this notion, it is important to consider, also, the theory of existentialism, for which Sartre was famous. Existentialism, as an approach to philosophy, may be encapsulated by Sartre's famous epigram that 'existence comes prior to essence' (Sartre 1973). In order to understand this, it may be useful to look at an example that Sartre himself uses. If we consider a man-made object such as a paper-knife, we can realise that before it came into existence, someone sat down and designed it. For the paper-knife, then, its 'essence' came prior to its 'existence': before it was made, someone had a fair idea of what it was going to be for. Sartre argues that, for people, exactly the opposite is true. First of all we exist, then *we create* our essence. Thus there is no one 'designing' us before we exist: we start from nothing and then we are responsible for what we become.

Contained in Sartre's argument is the notion that people are (psychologically at least) free to choose how they view themselves and the world. The temptation, very often, is for people to blame the past, other people or circumstances for how they are today. Whilst these factors clearly have an influence, what Sartre is saying is that today the individual decides for himself: he can *choose* to blame the past or circumstances, but that does not change his personal responsibility for decision-making. A person is what he makes himself. Clearly, as we have noted, this is a *psychological* freedom – it is a freedom of thought. We cannot exercise a similar *physical or social* freedom. It would be ludicrous, for instance, to argue that a person could choose to be seven feet tall or that he could choose the social circumstances into which he was born! The point Sartre makes is that, given these physical and social limitations, people make their own destiny.

It may be noted at this point that whilst Sartre's view of existentialism is atheistic, this need not necessarily be the case. Other commentators have argued for a Christian existentialism (e.g. Macquarrie 1966): whilst God is the prime mover, it is man who has to decide his own future and make his own decisions. In this version, man has been given 'free will' by God; in Sartre's version, God does not exist: man has free will anyway.

The second issue is the individual's *responsibility* for his life and his decision-making. A person cannot be *free* and yet not reponsible. Imagine, for instance, that I say: 'I am free to get married and I have chosen to do so, but the decision is really my parents'!' Such a statement is plainly illogical. Clearly, if I am free to choose, I cannot make another person responsible for my choice, since otherwise no such 'choice' exists.

These factors have important repercussions for ethical and professional decision-making. If Sartre's position is accepted (and it may not be), then the responsibility for *all* decisions rests squarely with the individual.

It may be worth considering to what degree nursing situations can be clarified through an appeal to situational ethics. Clearly, in many situations the nurse is dependent upon others to share in making decisions. Nor may we be keen to take on board Sartre's notion of total responsibility.

Such arguments can, however, make the nurse aware of how important ethical and behavioural decisions are and how important it is for her to shoulder responsibility. Such argument can also awaken nurses to the importance of considering the *context* of ethical decision-making. Whilst the Code of Conduct can be used as a guide to such decisions, it must also be borne in mind that *this* situation, for *this* person, is unique. It is necessary to remain flexible and open-minded and, where possible, come to each situation afresh. In weighing up the pros and cons of any situation and relating them to prior experience and knowledge, it must also be acknowledged how *different* this new situation is.

Perhaps, however, Sartre's position is a little black and white. It may be argued that many ethical and professional decisions are made by considering the evidence and comparing that evidence with previous situations that have occured and with which *this* situation may be compared. Out of this consideration and reflection on past experience arises the 'new' decision. An example may be useful here. If a nurse manager is attempting to make an important decision about how best to advise a member of staff she may well reflect back on previous situations which mirror this one, consider the 'unique' features of the present situation and look for some sort of 'fit' between past and present experience. Out of this balanced view, the manager makes her decision. In one sense, she is, of course, alone in making that decision. In another sense, however, she has considerable precedent in terms of her own and other people's past experience, on which to draw. Decision are never made in isolation. As has been discussed throughout this book, they arise out of a wide range of cultural, social, psychological and personal contexts. Perhaps, then, 'unique' situations are not as unique as they first appear!

One particular theme has recurred frequently throughout this book: the notion of the 'golden rule'. This is usually expressed as the idea that we should treat others as we ourselves would wish to be treated. This would seem to be a necessary requirement of anyone who makes ethical and professional decisions. The notion marks out the importance of fundamental human considerations: respect for others, consideration of the possible consequences of action, the need, always, to treat people as subjects and never as objects. Without such fundamental considerations, it seems difficult to see how any notion of ethical or professional decisions can begin to be made. It is notable, however, that even the 'golden rule' has its limitations. It may work well enough all the time that the individual is a thoughtful, caring person who wishes, himself, to be treated that way. It does not account for the person who does not *care* how he is treated! In this case, clearly, the notion of treating others as you would wish to be treated, does not apply! Christians would, of course, quote a higher authority for this type of action – the words of Jesus, 'This is my commandment, that ye love one another. . .' (John 15: 12).

This book has offered a variety of ways of addressing ethical and professional issues. The subject is a complex one and we hope that the book has raised more questions than it has answered. There cannot be a ready guide to the sorts of issue discussed, nor can there be a consensus on how to make decisions. What all ethical and professional decisions require is a firm grasp of as many of the facts as possible, an understanding of the various philosophical and theoretical ways of addressing problems of this nature, plus a certain courage and determination to *make* decisions. This is true throughout the field of nursing, from nurse learner to the most senior administrator or educator. Nursing is necessarily about decision-making. It is hoped that this book has helped in this process.

REFERENCES

Hall, C. (1954) *A Primer of Freudian Psychology.* Basic Books: New York.
Macquarrie, J. (1966) *Studies in Christian Existentialism.* S C M : London.
Sartre, J-P. (1956) *Being and Nothingness: an essay on phenomenological ontology* (Trans. H. Barnes): Philosophical Library: New York.
Sartre, J-P. (1973) *Existentialism and Humanism* (Trans. P. Mairet). Methuen: London.

BIBLIOGRAPHY

Recommended and Further Reading

Aroskar, M.A. (1980a) Anatomy of an ethical dilemma: the theory, the practice. *American Journal of Nursing* **80**: 4, 658-63.

Aroskar, M.A. (1980b) Ethics of nurse-patient relationships. *Nurse Educator* **5**: 2, 18-20.

Austin R. (1978) Professionalism and the nature of nursing reward. *Journal of Advanced Nursing* **3**: 19-23.

Baly, M. (1980) *Nursing and Social Change*. Heinemann: London.

Baly, M. (1983) Based on trust. *Nursing Mirror* **156**:12,33-34.

Baly, M. (1984) *Professional Responsibility*. Wiley: Chichester.

Barnes, H.E. (1967) *An Existential Ethics*. Knopf: New York.

Bartley, W.W. (1971) *Morality and Religion*. Macmillan: London.

Beardshaw, V. (1981) *Conscientious Objectors at Work*. Social Audit Ltd: London.

Beauchamp, T.L. and Walter, L. (1978) *Contemporary Issues in Bioethics*. Dickenson: Encino, California.

Beck, C.M., Crittenden, B.S. and Sullivan, E.V. (eds) (1971) *Moral Education*. Toronto University Press: Toronto.

Benjamin, M. and Curtis, J. (1981) *Ethics in Nursing*. OUP: New York.

Bergman, R. (1976) Evolving ethical concepts for nursing. *International Nursing Review* **23**: 4, 116-17

Berry, C. (1987) *The Rites of Life: Christians and Bio-Medical Decision Making*. Hodder and Stoughton: London.

Blackham, H.J. (1968) *Humanism*. Pelican: Harmondsworth.

Blomquist, C., Veatch, R.M. and Fenner, D. (1975) The teaching of medical ethics. *Journal of Medical Ethics* **1**:2, 96-103.

Bluglass, R. (1983) *A Guide to the Mental Health Act 1983*. Churchill Livingstone: Edinburgh.

Bok, S. (1980) *Lying: Moral Choice in Public and Private Life*. Quartet: London.

Brazier, M. (1987) *Medicine, Patients and the Law*. Pelican: Harmondsworth.

British Medical Association (1980) *Handbook of Medical Ethics*. BMA: London.

Broad, C.D. (1930) *Five Types of Ethical Theory*. Routledge and Kegan Paul: London.

Buber, M. (1937) *I and Thou*. T. and T. Clark: Edinburgh.

Bullock, A. and Stallybrass, O. (eds) (1977) *The Fontana Dictionary of Modern Thought*. Fontana: London.

Bunzl, M. (1986) A note on nursing ethics in the U.S.A. *Journal of Medical Ethics* **1** :4, 184.

Burnard, P. (1987) Spiritual distress and the nursing response: theoretical considerations and counselling skills. *Journal of Advanced Nursing* **12**, 377-382.

Campbell, A.V. (1984a) *Moral Dilemmas in Medicine*. Churchill Livingstone: Edingburgh.

Campbell, A.V. (1984b) *Moderated Love*. SPCK: London.

Campbell, A.V. and Higgs, R. (1982) *In that Case*. Darton, Longman and Todd: London.

Chapman, C.M. (1977) Concepts of Professionalism. *Journal of Advanced Nursing* **2**, 51-55.

Christie, R.J. and Hoffmaster, C.B. (1986) *Ethical Issues in Family Medicine*. OUP: New York.

Churchill, L. (1977) Ethical issues of a profession in transition. *American Journal of Nursing* **77**:5, 873-875.

Clay, T. (1987) *Nurses: Power and Politics*. Heinemann: London.

Committee of Enquiry into Human Fertilisation and Embryology: The Warnock Report (1984) HMSO: London.

Cook, J. (1987) *Whose Health is it Anyway?* New English Library: Sevenoaks, Kent.

Cox, C. (1979) Who Cares? Nursing and Sociology: the development of a symbiotic relationship. *Journal of Advanced Nursing* **4**, 237-252.

Davis, A.J. and Aroskar, M.A. (1983) *Ethical Dilemmas and Nursing Practice*. Appleton-Century-Crofts: Norwalk, Connecticut.

Dewey, J. (1966) *Democracy and Education*. The Free Press: New York.

Downie, R.S. and Calman, K.C. (1987) *Healthy Respect: Ethics in Health Care*. Faber and Faber: London.

Doxiadis, S. (ed.) (1987) *Ethical Dilemmas in Health Promotion*. Wiley: Chichester.

Drucker, P. (1977) *People and Performance*. Harper's College Press: New York.

Duncan, A.S., Dunstan, G.R. and Welbourne, R.B. (1981) *Dictionary of Medical Ethics*. Darton, Longman and Todd: London.

Dunlop, M.J. (1986) Is a science of caring possible? *Journal of Avanced Nursing* **11**, 661-670.

Dunstan, G.R. (1974) *The Artifice of Ethics*. SCM, London.

Dunstan, G.R. and Seller, M.J. (eds) (1983) *Consent in Medicine*. King Edward's Hospital Fund: London.

Durkheim, E. (1961) *Moral Education*. The Free Press: Glencoe, Ill.

Ededel, A. (1955) *Ethical Judgement*. The Free Press: Glencoe, New York.

Etzioni, A. (1969) *The Semi-Professions and Their Organisation.* Free Press: New York.

Evans, B. (1984) *Freedom to Choose.* The Bodley Head: London.

Faulder, C. (1985) *Whose Body is It? The Troubling Issue of Informed Consent.* Virago: London

Ferguson, M. and Turner, V. (1976) The dilemma of professionalism and Nursing Organisation. *Nursing Mirror.* 16 December.

Fletcher, J. (1955) *Morals and Medicine.* Gollancz: London.

Fletcher, J. (1967) *Moral Responsibility: Situation Ethics at Work.* SCM Press: London.

Frankena, W.K. (1973) *Ethics.* Prentice Hall: Englewood Cliffs, New Jersey.

Friedson, E. (1976) The Future of Professionalism. In Stacey et al. (1977) *Health and the Division of Labour.* Croom Helm: London..

Fromm, E. (1976) *To Have or To Be?* Abacus: London.

Gardner, R.F.R. (1977) *By What Standard?* Christian Medical Federation: London

General Medical Council (1983) *Professional Conduct and Discipline; Fitness to Practice.* GMC: London.

Gillon, R. (1986) *Philosophical Medical Ethics.* Wiley: Chichester.

Gostin, L. (1983) *A Practical Guide to Mental Health Law.* Mind Publications: London.

Griffin, A.P. (1983) A philosophical analysis of caring in nursing. *Journal of Advanced Nursing* **8**, 289-295

Grove, A. (1983) *High Output Mangement.* Souvenir Press: London.

Haring, B. (1974) *Medical Ethics.* St Paul Publications: Slough.

Harmin, M, Kirschenbaum, H. and Simon, S. (1973) *Clarifying Values Through Subject Matter.* Winston Press: Minneapolis.

Harris, J. (1986) *The Value of Life: An introduction to medical ethics.* Rouledge and Kegan Paul: London.

Hirst, P.H. (1974) *Moral Education in a Secular Society.* University of London Press: London.

Horan, F. and Jackson, V. (1984) Abortion: who decides? *Nursing Times* **80**: 10, 16-18.

Hoy, R. and Robbins, (1979) *The Profession of Nursing.* McGraw-Hill: London.

Hudson, W.D. (1970) *Modern Moral Philosophy.* Macmillan: London.

Hume, D. (1777) *Enquiry Concerning the Principles of Morals.* ed. L.A. Selby-Bigge, (1902). Clarendon: Oxford.

Hyde, A. (1976) The phenomenon of caring. *Nursing Research Report* **11**:3, 2 and 19.

Hyland, M. and Frapwell, C. (1986) Professional standards: Rough justice. *Nursing Times.* **82**:41, 32.

International Council of Nurses (1973) *Code of Nursing Ethics.* ICN: Geneva.

Jackson, D.M. (1972) *Professional Ethics: Who makes the rules?* CMF Publications: London.

Jameton, A. (1984) *Nursing Practice: the Ethical Issues.* Prentice-Hall: New Jersey.

Jarvis, P. (1977) Some comments on the RCN Code of Professional Conduct. *Nursing Mirror* **145**:47, 27-28.

Jarvis, P. (1983) *Religiosity: a theoretical analysis of the human response to the problem of meaning*. Institute for the Study of Worship and Religious Architecture, *Research Bulletin* : 51-66.

Johnson, M. (1983) Ethics in nurse education: a comment. *Nurse Education Today* **3**, 58-59.

Jupe, M. (1987) Ethics and Nursing Practice. *Senior Nurse* 7:3, 49-51

Kemp, J. (1970) *Ethical Naturalism*. Macmillan: London.

Kennedy, I. (1981) *Unmasking Medicine*. Allen and Unwin: London.

Kirschenbaum, H. (1977) *Advanced Values Clarification*. University Associates: La Jolla, California.

Kitson, A.L. (1987) A comparative analysis of lay caring and professional caring relationships. *International Journal of Nursing Studies* **24**:2, 155-165.

Kleinig, J. (1985) *Ethical Issues in Psychosurgery*. Allen and Unwin: London.

Leninger, M.M. (ed.) (1981) *Caring: An Essential Human Need*. Slack: Thorofare, New Jersey.

Levine, M. (1977) Ethics: nursing ethics and the ethical nurse: *American Journal of Nursing* **77**: 5, 845-849.

Lewin, K. (1952) *Field Theory and Social Change*. Tavistock: London.

McGilloway, O. and Myco, F (eds) (1985) *Nursing and Spiritual Care*. Harper and Row: London.

Magee, B. (1978) *Men of Ideas: Some Creators of Contemporary Philosophy*. BBC: London.

Mayeroff, M. (1972) *On Caring*. Harper and Row: New York.

Melia, K. (1984) Cracking the new code. *Nursing Times* **80**: 43, 20.

Meyers, D.W. (1970) *The Human Body and the Law*. Edinburgh University Press: Edinburgh.

Mill, J.S. (1867) *Utilitarianism*. Longmans: London.

Mill, J.S. (1910) *Utilitarianism, Liberty and Representative Government*. Dent: London.

Moore, D. (1987) The buck stops with you. *Nursing Times* **83**: 39, 54-56.

Moore, G.E. (1903) *Principia Ethica*. Cambridge University Press: London.

Morris, C. (1956) *Varieties of Human Value*. University of Chicago Press: Chicago.

Neuberger, J. (1987) *Caring for People of Different Faiths*. Austin Cornish: London.

Niblett, W.R. (1963) *Moral Education in a Changing Society*. Faber and Faber: London.

Nightingale, F. (1974) *Notes on Nursing: what it is and what it is not*, new edition. Blackie: London.

NUPE Wales Division (1985) *Dignity or Despair?* A Report on Care of the Elderly in Wales.

Papper, S. (1983) *Doing Right: Everday Medical Ethics*. Little, Brown: Boston.

Partridge, K.B. (1978) Nursing values in a changing society. *Nursing Outlook* **26** : 6, 356-360.

Patka, F. (ed.) (1972) *Existential Thinkers and Thought*. Citadel Press: Secaucus, New Jersey.

Paton, H.J. (1969) *The Moral Law: Kant's Groundwork of the Metaphysics of Morals*. Hutchinson: London.

Pearson, M. (1985) *Equal Opportunity in the N.H.S. – A Handbook*. Health Education Council and the National Extension College for Training in Health and Race: Cambridge.

Phillips, M. and Dawson, J. (1985) *Doctors' Dilemmas: Medical Ethics and Contemporary Science*. Harvester Press: Brighton, Sussex.

Pyne, R. (1987) A professional duty to shout. *Nursing Times*. **83**:42, 30-31.

Pyne, R. (1980) *Professional Discipline in Nursing*. Blackwell: London.

RCN (1976) *Code of Professional Conduct – a Discussion Document*. RCN: London.

RCN (1977) *Ethics Related to Research in Nursing*. RCN: London.

RCN (1979) *Charter and Byelaws*. RCN: London.

Ramsey, P. (1965) *Deeds and Rules in Christian Ethics*. Cambridge University Press: Cambridge.

Ramsey, P. (1978) *Ethics at the Edges of Life: Medical and Legal Intersections*. Yale University Press: New Haven, Connecticut.

Ramsey, P. (1970) *The Patient as Person: Explorations in Medical Ethics*. Yale University Press: New Haven, Connecticut.

Reader, W.J. (1966) *Professional Men*. Weidenfeld and Nicolson: London.

Reich, W.T. (1978) *Encyclopedia of Bioethics*. Macmillan: London.

Reiser, S.J., Dyck, A.J. and Curran, W.T. (1977) *Ethics in Medicine*. MIT Press: Boston.

Roach, M.S. (1984) *Caring, the Human Mode of Being, Implications for Nursing*. University of Toronto.

Robb, B. (1967) *Sans Everything*. Nelson: London.

Rogers, C.R. (1977) *On Personal Power*. Constable: London.

Rumbold, G. (1986) *Ethics in Nursing Practice*. Baillière Tindall: London.

Salvage, J. (1985) *The Politics of Nursing*. Heinemann: London.

Sampson, C. (1982) *The Neglected ethic: Religious and Cultural Factors in the Care of Patients*. McGraw-Hill: London.

Sarason, S.B. (1985) *Caring and Compassion in Clinical Practice*. Jossey Bass: San Franciso.

Sartre, J-P. (1973) *Existentialism and Humanism* (Trans. P. Mairet). Methuen: London.

Schrock, R. (1980) A Question of Honesty in Nursing Practice. *Journal of Advanced Nursing* **5** :2; 135-148.

Schulman, E.D. (1982) *Intervention in Human Services: A Guide to Skills and Knowledge*, 3rd Edition. C.V. Mosby: St Louis, Toronto.

Scrivenger, M. (1987) Ethics, Etiquette and the Law. *Nursing Times*. **83**:42, 28-29.

Scorer, G. and Wing, A. (eds) (1979) *Decision Making in Medicine: the practice of its ethics*. Arnold: London.

Scott, R. (1981) *The Body as Property*. Viking Press: London.

Sedgwick, P. (1982) *Psycho Politics*. Pluto Press: London.

Sieghart, P. (1985) Professions as the conscience of society. *Journal of Medical Ethics* **11** : 3, 117-122.

Simmons, D. (1982) *Personal Valuing: an Introduction*. Helson Hall: Chicago.

Simon, S.B., Howe, L.W. and Kirschenbaum, H. (1978) *Values Clarification: A Handbook of Practical Strategies for Teachers and Students*. A. and W. Visual Library: New York.

Steele, S.M. and Harmon, V.M. (1983) *Values Clarification in Nursing.* Appleton-Century-Crofts: Norwalk, Connecticut.
Stephenson, M. and Moran, L. (1987) The dilemma of ethics. *Senior Nurse* 7:3, 47-48.
Styles, M.M. (1982) *On Nursing : Towards a new endowment.* C.V. Mosby: St Louis.
Tate, B.L. (1977) *The Nurses Dilemma : Ethical Considerations in Nursing Practice.* ICN Code: Geneva.
Thiroux, J.P. (1980) *Ethics, Theory and Practice.* Glencoe Publishing: Encino, California.
Thompson, I.A., Melia, K. and Boyd, K. (1983) *Nursing Ethics.* Churchill Livingstone: Edinburgh.
Thompson, I.E. et al. (1981) Research Ethical Committees in Scotland. *British Medical Journal* **282**, 718-720.
Thomson, W.A.R. (1977) *A Dictionary of Medical Ethics and Practice.* Wright: Bristol.
Tillich, P. (1963) *Morality and Beyond.* Harper and Row: London.
Toulmin, S. (1958) *The Place of Reason in Ethics.* Cambridge University Press: Cambridge.
Townsend, P. and Davidson, N. (1982) *Inequalities in Health.* Penguin: Harmondsworth.
Tschudin, V. (1986) *Ethics in Nursing: the Caring Relationship.* Heinemann: London.
UKCC (1984) *Code of Professional Conduct.* UKCC: London.
Veatch, R.M. (1977) *Case Studies in Medical Ethics.* Harvard University Press: Cambridge, Mass.
Vousden, M. (1987) Top secret code? *Nursing Times* **83**:42, 25-27.
Warnock, M. (1970) *Existentialism.* Oxford University Press: London.
Watson, J. (1979) *Nursing: The Philosophy and Science of Caring.* Little, Brown: New York.
Watson, J. (1985) *Nursing: Human Science and Human Care: A theory of nursing.* Appleton-Century-Crofts: Norwalk, Connecticut.
White, R. (1985) *Political Issues in Nursing.* Wiley: Chichester.
Williams, B. (1976) *Morality: An Introduction to Ethics.* Cambridge University Press: Cambridge.
World Health Organisation – *Health Aspects of Human Rights with Special Reference to Developments in Biology and Medicine.* WHO: Geneva.
World Medical Association (1964) *Declaration of Helsinki.*
World Medical Association (1968) *Declaration of Sydney.*
Wright, D. (1971) *The Psychology of Moral Behaviour.* Penguin: Harmondsworth.
Young, A.P. (1981) *Legal Problems in Nursing Practice.* Harper and Row: London.

Index